THE INFERTILITY COMPANION

THE
INFERTILITY
COMPANION

HOPE AND HELP FOR COUPLES
FACING INFERTILITY

SANDRA L. GLAHN, TH.M. &
WILLIAM R. CUTRER, M.D.

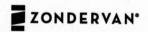

ZONDERVAN

Christian Medical Association
Resources

ZONDERVAN.com/
AUTHORTRACKER
follow your favorite authors

ZONDERVAN

The Infertility Companion
Copyright © 2004 by Sandra L. Glahn and William R. Cutrer

Requests for information should be addressed to:

Zondervan, *Grand Rapids, Michigan 49530*

Library of Congress Cataloging-in-Publication Data

Glahn, Sandra, 1958–
        The infertility companion : hope and help for couples facing infertility / Sandra L. Gahn and
    William R. Cutrer.
            p. cm.
        Includes bibliographical references and index.
        ISBN 978-0-310-24961-0 (softcover)
        1. Infertility—Religious aspects—Christianity. 2. Infertility—Psychological aspects.
    I. Cutrer, William, 1951-. II. Title.
    RC889.G536   2004
    248.8'6196692—dc22
    2004004099

Interior design by Michelle Espinoza

Printed in the United States of America

*For the patients who treasure human life in its earliest,
most vulnerable form above the fulfillment of their own God-given
yearnings, and for those who walk with them—Habakkuk's Hope,
Hannah's Prayer, agencies assisting with embryo adoption, and the
courageous physicians who value the dignity of life in God's image.*

CONTENTS

ACKNOWLEDGMENTS

It has been said that one who writes a book gives a part of one's self. *The Infertility Companion* is certainly such a work. It is the fruit of nearly forty combined years of exploring the medical, emotional, spiritual, relational, and ethical crisis of infertility.

We acknowledge with appreciation the many men and women we've met in doctors' offices and hospitals, at support group meetings, in churches, and at our conferences, who have entrusted to us the stories of their heartaches and victories. We are especially grateful to those who gave us permission (often enthusiastically) to retell their stories so that others might be helped by what they had experienced.

We are deeply indebted to Dr. Gene Rudd, of the Christian Medical Association, without whose counsel, encouragement, advocacy, and feedback this book would have been impossible.

We are also grateful to Dr. Steven Nakajima, of Louisville, Kentucky, for his input on medical information; to Keith Yates for providing the medical drawings; and for our readers and editors Jane Cutrer, Rose Courtney, Kathe Wunnenberg, Julie Watson, Cindy Lambert, Jane Haradine, Dr. Thomas Beam, Brian Phipps, Elizabeth Oates, and Dr. Sam E. Alexander, who have provided valuable feedback.

Finally, we are grateful to our spouses, Gary Glahn and Jane Cutrer, for their sacrificial love, unwavering support, and indispensable partnership in this ministry.

Chapter 1

Where We've Been

Your Companions in "the Ditch"

Sandi's Journey: Knots and Tangles

I am Sandra, daughter of Ann, daughter of Velma, daughter of Ella, all the way back to Eve. But the genes carried down through my ancestors will stop with me.

When I was a little girl, I never dreamed that I might be unable to have children. In my childhood home in Oregon's Willamette Valley, by mid-April the plum trees had sprouted purple blossoms and the whole world seemed to bloom with new life. Foals, calves, and lambs appeared in the fields. By Mother's Day, everything had either given birth or was celebrating hope, and I assumed that I would someday join in that process.

I was the fourth of five children. When I reached adolescence and started babysitting—which I loved—I became increasingly aware that many people have more children than they anticipate. I figured that, if anything, I'd fall into that group.

Fast-forward to age twenty-seven. My adoration of spring turned to dread as I felt out of sync with the rest of the world. While everything around me celebrated new life, I experienced spring more as an injury— almost as an indictment. With tear-stained cheeks, I watched birds build nests and lay eggs in our trees and thought of how children described me as "nobody's mommy." Mother's Day—that dreaded "M-Day"— came as the crowning insult.

My husband, Gary, and I had been married seven years, and he was starting his last year of seminary training (master's degree) in Dallas, Texas. In addition to our jobs—he at a law firm, I as a writer at an insurance company—and his studies, we served as part-time staff at our church, ministering to college students. After working full-time to put my husband through graduate school, I dreamed of quitting my job and staying home to take care of our children. Friends and family were asking when we'd start having babies, and it was finally time to get an "all clear" from my physician.

Dr. Bill Cutrer, my medical doctor, was also a seminary student, and he had a reputation for being a godly man with technical expertise. So I made the new-patient appointment, and after our consultation, he told me everything looked great. The next six months were wonderful. There's something magical about making love with the expectation that you'll produce something as marvelous as a child. The plans and dreams arrived in full force. I mentally picked out nursery colors. For graduation we got a car—a new station wagon big enough for the family we were going to have. I told a few close friends we were trying. We saved up all we could for the day when I could quit work.

Nine months passed with no success. I had expected to get pregnant the first month, but I told myself we'd been too busy. Then months turned into a year. But I wasn't too worried.

Another six months passed, though less quickly, and my sister confided to me that she was going through fertility testing. A pang of concern started gnawing inside me. Mary recommended a book about infertility, and I read it. Afterward I wrote in my journal, "The infertility fear is getting greater. There's a lot of denial on my part. I'm finally having to come to grips with the fact that there's a problem." I cried for the first time when someone asked when we were going to start a family. Three days later I wrote, "I'm facing that we may not have kids. It's tough. But his mercies *are* there, too." A church in British Columbia interviewed Gary by phone for a pastoral position. A week later I wrote in my journal, "My strong preference would be to stay in my current job until I know I can have kids. The Lord knows."

The job didn't pan out, and we both kept working. After eighteen months had passed, I returned to see Dr. Cutrer for what was supposed to be a belated annual checkup. All went fine until near the end, when he asked me a few questions.

"I think I just need to relax," I told him. "We've been trying to get pregnant, but we've probably been too busy to hit it right."

Looking up with gentle eyes, he rolled closer. "How long have you been trying?"

"About eighteen months." I had believed the myth so many people had told me: "Just relax and you'll get pregnant."

He spoke in a soothing tone. "No. Perhaps it's time to stop 'just relaxing.' There are a few simple things we can try. The pace is up to you." We could take it fast or slow, he told me, starting with the easiest, simplest test: a semenalysis on my husband.

Not a chance. *We're not infertile!* I thanked him politely and left for another eighteen months.

Threads of Grief

The time passed with increasing emotional pain. It got harder to deny the reality. So I finally returned to the doctor. By that time, I had heard a lot more about "Dr. Bill," as many of his patients called him:

"He stayed up with us all night rather than rush a C-section."

"He came in on the weekend to do our insemination."

"He prayed with us during our rough delivery."

Dr. Bill had a reputation for being a kind and compassionate man of God. I wish I could say we hit it off from the start, but at the time, I resented what I perceived as "doctor worship" on the part of many of his patients, so I determined to be distant.

Gary and I decided to begin the testing process. Dr. Bill began by testing Gary, who appeared to have no problem. Then Dr. Bill ran a lot of blood tests and did some studies to make sure I was ovulating. After that, I had an endometrial biopsy. I began to read everything I could find on the subject of infertility because through knowledge I felt empowered.

My sister called to say she'd had a laparoscopy (the so-called Band-Aid surgery) and her doctor had found endometriosis. Because there is sometimes a familial connection, Dr. Bill recommended that I, too, have a laparoscopy. But he also thought I might have a congenital structural problem. The day he told me that, I drove back to my office, shut the door, and sobbed my heart out. The shock of the news hit like a tsunami. *I really might never have children.*

I experienced a spiritual crisis. I had to face the fact that I had a mistaken perception of God. My life had gone fairly well up to that point, and I thought it might have something to do with my obedience. I secretly believed that if I continued feeding my "quarters" of obedience into God's cosmic vending machine, I'd get what I wanted. When that didn't happen, I realized that either something was wrong with my behavior or, the more helpless option, that God doesn't necessarily stick to such clear cause-and-effect arrangements. If the latter was the case, as I began to suspect it was, no amount of obedience would solve my fertility problem.

I wrote in my journal, "Waiting. Waiting. More waiting. I can hardly think of anything else. It was easy not to think about it when I wasn't facing the doctor or my charts every day or week, but it's hard to get it off my mind now that I'm constantly confronted with it."

When I stood around talking with other women, I felt somewhat like an imposter. I was incomplete, not quite a part of them, having failed what I perceived as the true test of womanhood: the rite of motherhood.

Monthly we would watch my ovaries on the ultrasound screen to help us "time it right." And I began taking medication for a mild hormonal imbalance. We found ourselves paying for multiple medical bills, having quickly discovered that most insurance policies will cover the diagnosis of infertility but not its treatment.

Dr. Bill prescribed the low-tech ovulation inducer, clomiphene citrate (brand names: Clomid, Serophene, Milophene). Of all the medications I would take during treatment, Clomid made me the craziest. One afternoon when I went in for a sonogram, I sarcastically asked Dr. Bill, "Could you give me more Clomid? I'm only crying at mall openings."

He responded in the schooled "doctor voice" that he has since labeled "vocal anesthesia," "Being the rather sentimental soul that I am, I'd probably cry at mall openings, too."

"I don't mean grand openings," I snapped. "I mean every day at ten when they open the doors."

Gary and I dreamed up a board game called "InFutility," which we patterned after Monopoly, except that instead of buying up real estate, the object was to get a child. We replaced the four railroads with roller coasters. Free parking was reserved for teens who got pregnant the easy way. "Community Test" cards were responses to people who made tacky comments, like the man who asked, "How can you miss something you never had?" We got to move ten spaces for quelling the urge to answer with, "You mean like your brain?" A little lame humor helped.

Then finally it happened. After three years of trying, I had a positive pregnancy test. But then I lost the pregnancy several days later. Soon after that, I had a difficult conversation with Dr. Bill. He told me he wanted to refer me to an endocrinologist. While I appreciated his desire that we find answers to my infertility, I had developed friendships with him and his staff, and I was actually starting to be nice to him. I had grown comfortable. Now I had to start over.

Threads of Patience

We called the endocrinologist and had to wait three months to get in. I became even more aware of how much of life is spent waiting.

I crossed off each calendar day leading up to my appointment. I wrote in my journal, "More opportunities for hope and despair ahead." When my brother-in-law told me I'd make a great mom, I wept. I realized then that I'd been wondering if the Lord was keeping me from being a mother because I'd be a failure at it.

During that time, our church asked us to start a support group for infertility patients, so Gary and I organized one. At the same time, I also served on the national board of a secular support organization for patients and providers. Their local chapter, on whose board I'd served, had been a lifeline. The group asked me to chair a medical symposium for patients, bringing together the state's top doctors and therapists. I said I would.

I had been told that infertility patients are second only to cancer patients in terms of what they will endure for a cure, and I found them to have a pretty high level of sophistication. I asked Dr. Bill to lecture on infertility and spirituality. He wondered if anyone would attend his workshop, but it ended up having the highest attendance of anything we offered.

Then I got pregnant again. Then lost the baby. Then again. Another loss. Pregnant. Loss. Pregnant. Loss. We experienced seven early pregnancy losses. Tests told us nothing. It was a mystery.

After seven years of trying to conceive, we watched as the odometer on our station wagon turned 100,000 miles. We'd stayed in Dallas to continue treatment. But we were getting to the point where it hurt more to go on than to quit. We were tired of it all. Then new tests suggested I had a rare immunological problem for which little could be done. So we took a year off to explore the possibility of never having children and devoting ourselves full time to ministry. Among other pursuits, we went with Dr. Bill and his wife, Jane, to Russia on a medical mission trip.

When we returned, I asked Dr. Bill to prescribe birth control pills. I wanted to stop mentally keeping track of my "cycle days," and I'd had enough pregnancy losses to know that my womb was not a safe place for a developing embryo. I needed to avoid conceiving.

At the end of that year, Gary and I learned that my immunological problem might be corrected with blood thinner and baby aspirin. So we pursued treatment again. It required giving myself daily shots in my thighs or stomach, and soon I was covered with bruises. Then I developed bleeding complications.

I finally reached my limit.

The next few weeks were filled with both mourning and resolution. I wrote: "Part of me wants to party and celebrate that we're through. But I will also grieve as the realization hits me. I feel unmotivated to work and tired from it all. But grief is a friend. I've learned to trust it to take me to the other side of emotional health."

I enrolled in some seminary classes to further my writing ministry. And we checked out U.S. adoption agencies. After the miscarriages, our infertility was pretty much public knowledge. We worked that to our advantage and recruited people to help us find a birth mother.

During the three years that followed, three birth mothers agreed to place their children with us and then changed their minds—either right before or on the day of birth.

How long, O LORD, how long? (Ps. 6:3).

Threads of Hope

"Don't send us any more birth mothers," we told our friends. "We don't think we could handle it." I wondered if I'd ever stop being suspicious that every piece of good news would turn into a disaster. I questioned whether my heart could ever freely love a child now.

Not long after that, I met with a book publisher about a fiction project. In the course of the conversation, I expressed my disappointment in how little helpful information I'd found in the Christian market about infertility—especially on the ethics of high-tech treatment—and he told me to send him a book proposal. I was stunned. I was a magazine writer; it had never crossed my mind to write a *book*.

After giving it some thought, I contacted Dr. Bill. It seemed that a book about infertility and pregnancy loss would have more credibility with a combination of perspectives. He agreed to work on the project with me. As he put it, a team of the two of us could be "doctor-patient, male-female, sane-insane." So we began to write.

The book gave me a constructive channel for my grief. When the odometer turned to 200,000 miles, Gary and I traded in the first station wagon for another. I pursued finishing my master's degree in theology, choosing to focus much of my research on infertility as a spiritual crisis. And finally, more than a year after we'd started, Dr. Bill and I finished the manuscript.

These activities opened doors to a writing and speaking ministry for me and for us as a team.

I know now that I will never give birth. You'll read snippets of Gary's and my story and our path to resolution throughout the book, though the whole picture of what was medically wrong and all of God's reasons for allowing it will remain mysteries to us.

Yet when I look back on where I have been and what the Lord has done, I can't help but think of a tapestry. For so long, the individual painful situations made no sense. I shook my head as I tried to figure out what God was doing with my life and wondered why he had allowed so much death—whether of embryos or dreams. But now that I reflect on the eighteen years since we started down the infertility path, I can see that each grief was like a colorful thread—gold for grace to endure marital stress, green for growth as we lamented through emotional upheaval, crimson for his arms beneath us when each period started. The Tapestry Maker was weaving a landscape. By itself, each thread meant nothing. Yet taken as a whole, it is plain to see that he was weaving a picture that tells a story—the story of his faithfulness in our lives.

The Weaver is making something beautiful of your life, too. It doesn't seem to make sense now, and parts of it will never make sense this side of eternity. You're in the midst of knots and tangles, looking at the incomplete picture from the back side. And there are no magic words to make the pain go away. But while you're there, being stretched on the Weaver's loom, know that *you are not alone.*

Dr. Bill's Journey

I (Dr. Bill) experienced my first deep personal connection with infertility when a patient arrived in the emergency room with a ruptured ectopic pregnancy. As the chief ob-gyn resident at Baylor Medical Center in Dallas, Texas, I worked with her infertility doctor to perform the needed surgery. In the follow-up days of her recovery, I observed this couple's pain. They were Christians who desperately wanted a baby. Sitting on the hospital bed with her husband holding her, the patient wept so hard that she could barely catch her breath and choke out "Why?" over the loss of their child.

Up to that point, I had given little thought to ectopic pregnancies as "children," because I was still thinking of pregnancy loss mostly as a medical condition, ignoring the emotional and spiritual ramifications of such a loss. I was trained in an atmosphere in which it was considered fine to have faith but unprofessional to bring it into the health-care arena. So my patients taught me a lot about spirituality and incorporating faith into medical care. These precious insights from those in the midst of their pain changed me and changed the way I would practice medicine.

A lot has happened since my early days as an ob-gyn in the 1970s. For more than three decades now, the treatment of infertility has been a passion of mine. In the beginning of my career, infertility was almost as prevalent as it is now, but our understanding of the causes was in its infancy, and few effective therapeutic regimens existed. Surgical techniques were just being developed, as was our understanding of endometriosis and pelvic inflammatory disease and their effects on pelvic architecture and fertility potential.

Doctors watched with anticipation the emergence of proper operative technique, microsurgical skills, various anti-inflammatory medications to prevent postoperative adhesions, the development of laparoscopy, and tools designed to do complex procedures through the scope as outpatient procedures. Those were exciting times, though we learned through bad experiences that some operative techniques actually impaired future fertility by causing more damage to the anatomy than they fixed. We worked to convince colleagues in various other surgical specialties that with any abdominal or pelvic surgery on a female patient, they should take future fertility into consideration.

Meanwhile the pharmaceutical armamentarium was expanding beyond "Clomid or more Clomid." Laboratory hormone evaluations became available. Doctors could test for and correct prolactin excess, androgen excess, abnormal estrogen-progesterone ratios, and low thyroid levels. Anatomic evaluation went well beyond the hysterosalpingogram and the "dinosaur" Rubins test to new scopes through which surgeons could evaluate not only pelvic structures such as the uterus, tubes, and ovaries but the inside of the uterus as well.

When we started working with laparoscopes and lasers, we realized we could do a lot to treat anatomical problems without the big operation and microscopes. Hysteroscopes went from the prototype "contact scopes" to useful operative scopes that could see inside the uterus and thus add to our understanding of anatomical issues stemming from congenital abnormalities or uterine fibroids. Now new, tiny scopes exist for seeing into the fallopian tubes themselves.

The momentum in the field of infertility increased with the Steptoe-Edwards announcement in 1978 of the first so-called test-tube baby. Fertility as a specialty began to take shape as a hybrid of gynecology and endocrinology. With the advent of more high-tech procedures and micromanipulation, clinics began to spring up, and competition for patients and dollars grew fiercer.

Immunological studies began to push their way onto the playing field, and the number of "undiagnosed infertility" cases began to shrink. Therapeutic approaches to each of the diagnoses uncovered by testing became better substantiated by case trials, enabling us to assist many couples in their quest for offspring.

From the doctor's side of the desk, I found the workup of the infertile couple to be both fascinating and exasperating. Even the most conscientious evaluation might yield no significant findings. Worse still was making an accurate diagnosis but having the therapeutic measures fail to bring about a live birth.

Millions of couples experience infertility, more than half of whom can expect successful outcomes with currently available treatment options. Some of the technologies used, however, push the ethical envelope. In fact, some of the procedures burst through the envelope. That we *can* do something medically does not necessarily mean we *should* do it.

Due to the many ethical considerations associated with treatment, infertility made its way into the bioethical arena. How far is too far? Should every couple use every available technology? What about the expense? Must a couple have children to be a family? These questions demanded answers.

From Health Care to Soul Care

I practiced medicine in Dallas from 1980 to 1994, and I enrolled in Dallas Theological Seminary (DTS) in 1985, anticipating a second career as a medical missionary. I wanted a better theological understanding of bioethical issues. My training at DTS was instrumental in helping me to see a pregnancy loss as the loss of a child, and I grew to better understand the profound spiritual implications of infertility. My training also helped me to clarify certain positions on medical intervention and approaches to fertility problems, and I became personally interested in bioethics—the morality of health-care issues.

But there remained much mystery. Why do some couples who appear perfectly suited for parenthood suffer with reproductive failure? Why do so many early pregnancies, precious tiny human lives, end in miscarriage? How do we meaningfully comfort and love those whose dream of bringing a child into the world—a good and godly dream— never comes to pass?

Motivated by the desire to understand and encourage couples in their longing to reproduce, I loved medical practice and still love the art of medicine. But as I concluded my seminary degree, health issues necessitated open-heart surgery for me and forced a shift in careers. While recuperating, I found myself transitioning into both a church ministry and a position with the Christian Medical and Dental Associations. This rewarding time allowed me to study further the ethical issues of medical care, even as the skills relating to infertility treatment were accelerating.

When I was in medical school, our professors taught us to "stay objective"—to remain distant so that the burdens of caring for people would not overwhelm us. I have never heeded this advice. I believe instead that infertile couples need caregivers who will enter into their lives and help them bear their pain.

Several years ago I was invited to join the faculty at the Southern Baptist Theological Seminary in Louisville, Kentucky. I accepted the position and teach classes in medical bioethics, pastoral care in human crises, spiritual formation, and marriage enrichment. Although Sandi and I now live nearly a thousand miles apart, we continue to write together and lead conferences to encourage infertile couples. I also devote specific time in my human crises class to training future ministers to care for those who struggle with infertility.

Today I have the privilege of serving as the medical director at A Woman's Choice Resource Center and as the director of the Gheens Center for Family Ministry. In that capacity, I sponsor Habakkuk's Hope, a support group on the seminary campus for infertile couples. The prophet Habakkuk foretold the invasion and desolation of his country, but he still rejoiced in God's sovereign purposes. Thus, the name of the support group is based on Habakkuk 3:17–19: "Though the fig tree does not bud and there are no grapes on the vines, though the olive crop fails and the fields produce no food, though there are no sheep in the pen and no cattle in the stalls, yet I will rejoice in the LORD, I will be joyful in God my Savior. The Sovereign LORD is my strength; he makes my feet like the feet of a deer, he enables me to go on the heights." Habakkuk's Hope was founded by a seminary student's wife whose own circumstances showed her the need for such a ministry. She and her husband sought to start a family but soon discovered that she had breast cancer. After completing cancer treatments, doctors told her, a woman of thirty-six at the time, that she would have to wait two years before attempting to have children. She quickly recognized how much a support group could help those suffering the pain of infertility and pregnancy loss. She and many like her have taken their pain and used it as a means to bless others.

Your Companions

One of my favorite "stories to live by" is about a farmer who is driving along and sees that his neighbor has accidentally driven a tractor into a ditch. The neighbor is hopelessly stuck. The farmer does not have a tow chain or a rope, so he does all that he can do—he gets out of his car, climbs into the cab of the tractor, and sits with his friend in the ditch.

Our desire and prayer is that through this *Infertility Companion*, we can provide some company and comfort in the ditch that is infertility.

As you can see, we have experienced the infertility struggle from a variety of angles. Sandi's perspective comes from having endured medical treatment, miscarriages, and failed adoptions and from leading support groups, serving on boards, teaching seminars, and concentrating her theological education on fertility-related issues.

I have sat on the other side of the desk (and the operating table) for infertility workups, surgeries, miscarriages, ectopic pregnancies, and crisis pregnancies leading to adoptions. I've led workshops, sponsored support groups, and taught pastoral counselors. One pastoral student of mine who has been through infertility aptly describes the trauma of being unable to have a child:

> We have not steadily been faith-filled or optimistic either toward God or life throughout this struggle. There have been wrenching pains, tear-filled nights, lost friends, confusion, frustration, awkward moments, expensive medical procedures, and tons of different emotions—guilt, doubt, anxiety and depression. We have wondered at God's sovereignty. We have felt guilt that perhaps we were facing God's judgment for past sins. We have expressed anger toward God. There have even been nights when we have contemplated leaving the faith and not looking back. The wounds we have felt at times have pierced so deeply that we wondered if we would survive at all. Certainly, if we were given a choice, we never would have chosen to walk down this road of infertility. Yet today we find ourselves with a deepened faith, a deepened love for one another, and a deepened belief that God works all things, even infertility, together "for good for those who love God and are called according to His purpose." We have experienced intense pain, and are now experiencing intense joy that God is sovereign and that He cares deeply for us. We are certain that His purposes for our sufferings are very good. We have not always been in this place and it has been a hard, pain-filled, grueling journey to arrive here.[1]

In the pages ahead, our desire is to walk with you, the reader, on the path through this treacherous journey called infertility. Our goal in writing *The Infertility Companion* is to point to the God of all comfort, who alone can minister to the needs of infertility patients and those seeking to assist them. We cannot take away the pain, but perhaps through sharing our own journeys and the knowledge we've gained, we can minister God's grace in "the ditch" and thus equip readers to face their heartbreak with renewed hope—an eternal hope that never disappoints (Rom. 5:5).

Note: Many infertile couples and individuals have shared their stories with us, hoping they might encourage our readers. We have included their quotes throughout the book, setting them in italics. At times we have combined or slightly altered their situations to protect identities or to fit in the allotted space. In addition, a few of the stories in the text and a small number of the italicized items come from our personal experiences, yet we may not always identify them as ours.

Chapter 2

The Wedded Unmother

Myths and Facts

"Just relax."

"It's all in your head."

"It's a woman's problem."

"You waited too long, honey."

No doubt you've heard them all. When it comes to fertility, it seems that everyone has an opinion, and "mis-conceptions" abound. Perhaps it's because so many people have a vested interest in the topic; nine in ten Americans who marry say they want at least one child.

Most fertility patients are educated consumers; they can correctly pronounce words such as "hysterosalpingogram," explain the difference between mobility and motility, and say words like "sperm" in a crowd without blushing. Sometimes, though, despite the abundance of available information, patients and those in their support networks end up with wrong ideas. So to make sure we all start out with the same foundational understanding, we'll begin by considering some of the more common misunderstandings and clearing some of them up with "Myths and Facts about Infertility."

Myth: Infertility is the same thing as sterility, and it's rather rare.

Fact: Sterility is the complete inability to reproduce; infertility is "subfertility," or impaired fertility. A sterile person cannot reproduce; about 65 percent of those who seek treatment for infertility will eventually go on to have a baby.[1] The World Health Organization (WHO) estimates that infertility affects more than 80 million people worldwide.[2] The American Society for Reproductive Medicine (ASRM) estimates that infertility affects 6.1 million American women and their partners,[3] which adds up to about 12.9 percent of married couples of reproductive age.[4]

Primary infertility is the inability to conceive after one year of unprotected intercourse for patients thirty-five years old or younger, or the inability to conceive in a six-month period for those in the over thirty-five age group. Infertility also includes the inability to carry a pregnancy to term.

Secondary infertility is defined as the inability to conceive or carry a child to term after one or more live births. An estimated 3 million U.S. couples suffer from secondary infertility, almost double the number in 1995.[5] While many people seek infertility treatment, not everyone who is infertile gets medical attention. About one-third of North American women experience fertility problems in their lifetime, but only about 44 percent of these women seek medical care. Younger women and women of higher socioeconomic status are more likely to seek medical assistance.[6] Women with secondary infertility are about half as likely to seek medical assistance as are women with primary infertility.[7]

According to a 1995 survey, 2 percent of American women of reproductive age—1.2 million women—had received medical advice or treatment for infertility within the previous year.[8] About 15 percent of women of childbearing age in the United States have at some point received an infertility service.[9]

The percentage of childless infertile couples in the U.S. has been on the rise, increasing from 14.4 percent in 1965 to 18.5 percent in 1995, according to the National Center for Health Statistics. Some of this increase is due to the aging of the baby boom generation and delayed childbearing.[10]

Infertility also includes miscarriage. Close to one million women in the United States experience pregnancy loss each year; many of these women are suffering at least their third consecutive pregnancy loss. Some experts say that up to half of all *actual* pregnancies end in miscarriage, because many losses occur before a woman realizes she is pregnant.[11] Others put this figure even higher, suggesting that as many as three-quarters of all fertilized eggs are lost.[12]

Myth: Women are having babies well into their forties, so it's probably safe to delay childbearing.

Fact: Fertility rates are definitely age related. Researchers used to say that the average woman's fertility dropped in her early thirties (with the big plunge after age thirty-five), but current studies suggest that, on average, female fertility begins its meaningful slide at age twenty-seven. It drops off more significantly around age thirty-five and drops dramatically at age forty. Thanks to vigorous exercise, a woman who is thirty-five may have the cardiovascular system of a woman in her twenties, yet her ovarian function is still that of a thirty-five-year-old.

Some women enter menopause prematurely, even in their twenties, while some maintain a fairly high level of fertility into their late thirties. Clinics that use ovum (egg) donors report dramatic differences in success rates when using egg donors in their twenties versus those in their forties. So as a rule, when it comes to fertility, younger is better. A woman desiring children after age thirty should feel free to seek medical help if conception doesn't occur within the first six months, sooner if she isn't cycling regularly. Though we read stories about women giving birth as much as three decades beyond this age, the mothers in such cases conceived using the eggs of a younger donor.

A woman under age thirty has a 20 percent chance of becoming pregnant in any given month, but when a woman is over forty, her odds plummet to 5 percent. She is born with about 300,000 eggs. But only a few thousand remain by the time she reaches her forties. Older eggs do not fertilize as easily as younger eggs, nor do they respond as well to reproductive hormones. They also have more chromosomal irregularities, resulting in a higher number of miscarriages and children with birth defects.[13] Women between the ages of thirty and thirty-nine receive the most fertility treatments.

What about men and aging? In the past few decades, the number of American men between the ages of thirty-five and fifty-four fathering children has increased by 25 percent.[14] So men, like women, are putting off having children. And many have that luxury: Pablo Picasso sired a child at sixty-six, Anthony Quinn at seventy-eight, and Tony Randall of *The Odd Couple* at seventy-six.[15] Strom Thurman fathered a child at eighty-one.[16] In contrast, no woman in modern history has conceived in her seventies or eighties—especially not with her own eggs. Yet while a woman's "biological clock" gets all the press, a man has one, too; it just ticks more slowly. The journal *Human Reproduction* reported that men's fertility starts declining after age thirty-five.[17]

Researchers at the University of Washington–Seattle examined sperm samples from sixty men between the ages of twenty-two and sixty. They found that the sperm cells of men over age thirty-five tended to have lower sperm motility, more damage to sperm cell DNA, and less natural elimination of damaged sperm. Apparently the longer a man lives, the more likely it is that environmental and behavioral factors, such as smoking, pesticides, exposure to certain chemicals, and alcohol use, will affect his sperm.[18] Perhaps as a result of these environmental factors, twenty-five-year-old women are more than twice as likely to have a miscarriage when their partners are thirty-five or older than when their partners are younger than thirty-five.[19]

Myth: Infertility is mostly a woman's problem.

Fact: A survey conducted by the British Broadcasting Corporation (BBC) found that more than two-thirds of people interviewed thought infertility was associated with a woman's fallopian tubes. A similar number of the 1,300 men and women interviewed did not realize that half of all infertility cases are caused by male problems.[20] The ASRM, stating that infertility affects men and women with almost equal frequency, puts it in rough terms: "About one-third of infertility cases can be attributed to male factors, and about one-third to factors that affect women. For the remaining one-third of infertile couples, infertility is caused by a combination of problems in both partners."[21] And as many as 20 percent of couples who have had complete workups are diagnosed with unexplained infertility because no specific cause is identified.[22]

It should come as no surprise that male fertility problems usually relate to urological problems, and female factors usually relate to ovulation. Abnormal sperm function is the major cause in one-third to one-half of all cases of male infertility, and the underlying problems are correctable about half the time. Male infertility is often easier to detect but more difficult to correct than female infertility. Normal sperm counts range from 20 million to 60 million cells per milliliter (one-fifth of a teaspoon) of semen, and anything below that means a low sperm count, though that does not necessarily mean a man can't biologically father a child. Other qualities (such as sperm form and motility) are also important. With procedures such as intracytoplasmic sperm injection (ICSI), in which a single sperm is injected into the egg, a much lower number of sperm is required than with natural reproduction.

Myth: Standing on your head after intercourse will improve your odds of conceiving.

Fact: If a woman stands on her head after intercourse, it will not improve her odds of conceiving. However, using a pillow to elevate her hips for about fifteen minutes may help the semen to contact the cervical mucus.

Myth: At least infertile couples are "having fun trying."

Fact: In a study of more than two thousand Christian women, "lengthy infertility treatment" was listed as one of the four key causes of sexual aversion. (The other three were childhood sex abuse, rape, and painful labor and delivery.)[23] Another study of "sexual satisfaction and functioning in patients seeking infertility treatment" suggested that "women undergoing infertility treatment experience significant changes in various aspects of sexual desire, arousal, orgasm, length of foreplay, and frequency of intercourse."[24]

Most couples report a decrease in the frequency of sexual relations after a diagnosis of infertility. What was once a source of emotional intimacy often becomes "love by the calendar," and infertile couples say they feel a loss of privacy, sometimes even envisioning a doctor in the room during sexual intimacy. Both male and female infertility patients report a decrease in their level of sexual satisfaction, with the women also reporting that they feel less comfortable with their sexuality. Infertile couples report sexual difficulties five times more often than do fertile couples. More than one infertility counselor has told us, "I've never seen a couple going through fertility treatment who felt they had a great sex life."

Myth: Infertility is caused by the need to relax. ("Just relax.")

Fact: Looking at the above statistics about the causes of infertility, we can see that about 80 to 85 percent of the time, doctors find a diagnosable medical cause, for which no amount of relaxation will help. And in cases of unexplained infertility, often the problem is due to a factor such as chromosomal abnormalities that are impossible to discover through a routine workup. (In other words, if a couple's infertility is said to be "unexplained," that does not mean psychological factors are the cause. A diagnosis of unexplained infertility may mean that there is no method yet developed for diagnosing the problem.)

Chronic stress and fatigue *do* alter hormones, but most fertility drugs can compensate in cases where hormones fall outside of normal ranges.

Those who tell fertility patients to "just relax" actually make it more difficult for them to do so. Infertility is more likely to *cause* stress than to *be caused by* stress. Some people will observe a woman who is focused on conceiving and determine that her infertility is caused by wanting children too much. Others see a woman who is career-focused and conclude that she lacks interest in children. (Her career may actually be her way of dealing with the grief and paying for the treatment.) Sadly, they assume she is "too into her career to make the sacrifices required to have children." It seems that no matter what she does, the woman is at fault, and "it's all in her wrong attitude."

Some people who frequently teach about infertility's strong mind-body connection have put together programs for helping couples conceive. Steps to success involve maintaining good health: couples should stop smoking, stop drinking, and bring their weights within normal ranges. These suggestions do enhance fertility in many cases. Note, however, that even those who see a strong mind-body link make recommendations for how to improve one's physical health, not just "mind-over-matter" recommendations.

Patients should be wary of expensive mind-body workshops that make unrealistic promises or boast of high success rates based on very small test groups. Questions to ask would include: Over what period of time did you have that success rate? What percentage of those patients took medications and did intrauterine inseminations (IUIs) during the same cycles they went through the program? And what percentage of those patients had unexplained infertility?

Anecdotal evidence always abounds: "Sleeping with crystals under the bed enhances fertility. I know this woman who . . ." or "Kicking back in Tahiti will do the trick. We know this couple who . . ." In our culture, the effectiveness of relaxation as a means for increasing the likelihood of conception has been enormously exaggerated and probably will continue to be. More research is needed with larger test groups to determine exactly how much of a mind-body connection exists. A controlled study examining pregnancy rates among those using only relaxation and nutrition approaches balanced against a similar group with parallel stress but electing not to use these approaches would be difficult to conduct, but such a study would be necessary to establish an incontrovertible link.

Myth: A woman must have an orgasm to conceive.

Fact: Approximately one in ten married women has never experienced an orgasm, and millions of these women have conceived. Additionally, many people believe that when a woman achieves climax—especially after the man does—fertility may be slightly increased due to enhanced sperm movement created by a small suction effect that's thought to pull sperm into the woman's uterus. There's a certain logic behind this theory. Yet while studies have shown that such a "vacuum effect" exists, whether it actually brings about a higher pregnancy rate is as of yet unproven.

Myth: Adoption cures infertility. ("Just adopt and you'll get pregnant.")

Fact: Of those adoptive families who have experienced infertility, approximately half have endured medical treatment for an average of three years prior to adopting.[25] It has been estimated that between 5 and 14 percent of couples who quit treatment and pursue adoption eventually go on to conceive.[26] That's about the same percentage as for couples who quit treatment, choose *not* to adopt, and subsequently conceive. The "just adopt" advice is a variation on the "just relax" theme. The idea behind it is that if couples stop thinking about getting pregnant, it will happen.

A woman who conceived after adopting told of how her doctor had found that she and her husband were passing an infection back and forth to each other, and a simple round of antibiotics cleared it up. Many people said to her, "See? You adopted and you got pregnant! Works every time!"

She said what she thought of such comments: "I smiled and nodded, thinking, 'No, if you want a clear cause-and-effect relationship, I took antibiotics and got pregnant. But since that's none of your business, think whatever you want.'"

Myth: You can always adopt. ("If you adopt, the pain will go away.")

Fact: Adoption is a wonderful solution for many couples, but it does not erase all the pain of infertility. In *Taking Charge of Infertility*, author Pat Johnston identifies six key losses stemming from infertility:

1. loss of control
2. loss of individual genetic continuity
3 loss of a jointly conceived child
4. loss of the pregnancy and birth experiences
5. loss of emotional gratification surrounding pregnancy and birth
6. loss of an opportunity to nurture and parent a new generation[27]

For some infertile couples, the greatest loss is the inability to participate in the wonder of creating a child together—a key loss not solved by adoption. In the book of Genesis, we read what happened right after Adam and Eve left the Garden of Eden. The text says, "Now the man had intimate relations with his wife, Eve, and she conceived and bore Cain, saying, 'I have created a man along with the Lord'" (Gen. 4:1, my translation).[28]

Imagine what it must have been like for Eve. Her body began to change form. Though she might have noticed pregnant animals, she must have wondered what was happening to her. She'd never seen a human baby. If she even suspected she was pregnant, she had no way of knowing her due date—no sonograms, weighings, urine tests. And even if she did realize she was pregnant, she might have wondered how that thing was going to come out of her!

But then, after a great deal of pain, she saw in the face of her son the reflection of her own humanity. After the agony of childbirth with no epidural or Lamaze preparation, Eve must have gazed at this tiny creature looking back at her through eyes that blended her features with Adam's. His nose, her mouth, her hair coloring, his ears—their passion for each other and the wonder of God's creation all working together in the form of a tiny body. It's no wonder that Eve exclaimed, "I've created an 'Adam' with the help of the Lord!" (Gen. 4:1, my translation).

Adoption is a wonderful solution for the desire to nurture and parent the next generation, the last of the six key losses author Johnston describes. Yet it doesn't "solve" the other losses. That's why "You can always adopt," said in response to an infertile couple's pain, is an insensitive, annoying suggestion. These couples are feeling the other key losses acutely. So by mentioning adoption as a pat answer, the would-be encourager totally invalidates the grief that runs through the very core of the infertile person. The suggestion that all the pain of infertility can be magically wiped away by adoption is clearly a simplistic answer to a complicated scenario.

Myth: Most infertile couples seek high-tech medical treatment.

Fact: Only about 10 percent of infertile couples seek assisted reproductive technologies (ARTs).[29] In fact, fewer than half of infertile American women even seek treatment, let alone high-tech treatment. The U.S. Centers for Disease Control estimates that ARTs account for approximately 1 percent of total births in the United States.[30]

The number of Christian couples pursuing high-tech treatment is probably much lower, because many Christians hesitate to seek even the simplest forms of infertility diagnosis and treatment out of concern that doing so might demonstrate a lack of faith.

Most couples in average- and lower-income groups can't afford high-tech treatment. Statistics show that high-tech infertility services are most often used by men and women who are Caucasian, college educated, older than thirty, in a higher-income bracket, and seeking to have their first biological child. While there is no significant association between race or ethnicity and infertility, there is a strong link between a couple's economic status and their ability to seek treatment.[31] Cultural differences related to body weight and other factors, however, can affect the outcomes of ARTs.[32]

Myth: Infertility is a curse from God.

Fact: The only clear connection between an individual's infertility and punishment from God, according to Old Testament law, was a pronouncement in the cases of adultery (Num. 5:20), including relations between a nephew and an aunt and between a brother-in-law and a sister-in-law. In those cases, the immoral couples would die childless (Lev. 20:20–21).

The fact that so many people today have difficulty conceiving is consistent with what God predicted long ago. When describing the consequences of sin in the Garden of Eden, the Hebrew text tells us, "God told the woman, 'I will greatly multiply your pain and your conception; in pain you shall bring forth children'" (my translation). The two words "pain" and "conception" appear to go together as one thought, similar to how we sometimes combine two nouns—sick and tired—to express one idea.

At the very least, the ancient text refers to the pain of human birth being increased. Interestingly enough, horses normally deliver within forty-five minutes. While they feel discomfort, it's nothing like the agony a human mother experiences in her twelve-hour-plus ordeal. Pain fibers surround the human cervix, yet doctors can stab it, cut it, or burn it with impunity. But when the cervix is stretched during labor, human pain is impressive.

Yet more than physical pain is probably implied in the Genesis account. The human difficulty with conception, pregnancy, and delivery are doubtless part of the overall consequences of the Fall. In fact, when we look around at all of creation, we see numerous other evidences of the world's "fallenness." This is *not* to say that an *individual infertile woman* is under some kind of specific curse. Rather, it suggests that we can lump infertility in with death, natural disasters, disease, broken relationships, injury, and weeds—processes that have affected us all since our first parents left Eden. (In chapters 6 and 7, we'll explore in-depth the myth that infertility is a curse from God.)

Myth: Doctors take huge risks with embryos in high-tech programs, making these options unethical.

Fact: When looking at ART cycles, we find that the statistics do little to help us to assess the actual risk taken with human life. So the above statement may be partially true, depending on whether the patients take a proactive role in managing their treatment.

A summary of 384 programs doing ART cycles in 2001 reported that 107,587 ART procedures resulted in 29,344 live births (deliveries of one or more living infants) and 40,687 babies.[33] Yet these figures do not tell us the ratio of *embryos* to live births; this ratio is not readily available.

A common misconception is that a 30 percent IVF success rate means that 70 percent of the embryos died, and that's not true. Take an in vitro fertilization (IVF) cycle in which no fertilization occurs and a cycle in which one embryo is created and carried to term, and you have a 50 percent success rate, even though 100 percent of the embryos were carried to term. In addition, even an unassisted menstrual cycle involves significant embryo risk, as in natural conceptions a high number of embryos die.

Patients can take a proactive role in managing their treatment by insisting that all attempts are made to minimize the risk to the embryo. It is possible to use ARTs without compromising a high view of life. For example, couples can limit the number of potential embryos (that is, the number of eggs exposed to sperm) to the number they are willing to carry to term in that cycle, thus avoiding the ethical minefield of pregnancy reduction. (We'll discuss this further in chapter 13.) Nevertheless, we will probably never see IVF clinics with high ratios of created embryos to live births because the more we learn about genetics, the more certain we become that a high percentage of embryos never make it past the one-cell (zygote) stage. That's probably not only because medicine has "messed with the process" but because the world—right down to the tiny human embryo—is quite fragile.

Scientists are currently working to improve the process of freezing and thawing human eggs. Once this process is perfected, we can more easily avoid some of the ethical disasters associated with creating multiple embryos and freezing some of them. At the time of this writing, about half of all embryos fail to survive the thawing process, a troubling statistic for those who value human life. Once we can freeze and thaw *eggs* without destroying any of their DNA, we can store gametes (eggs and sperm) rather than embryos. Then even if eggs have a poor survival rate, we won't have the moral dilemma associated with thawing human beings.

Yes, infertile couples encounter these myths everywhere, when they least expect them. We have listed here only the most common myths to show just how difficult infertility can be. And while these myths and others abound, there's one fact that all patients agree on: infertility treatment is hard stuff.

A writer for *Newsweek* described well some of the frustrations of a couple going through treatment: "First they live by the unbending rule of the calendar for conjugal relations on the prescribed three days of every month . . . even though it now brings them all the joy of taking out the trash. Then they become human pincushions, their rear ends sore from twice-a-day hormone shots that sometimes make their ovaries inflate to the size of baseballs. . . . They fume at insurers who regard infertility treatment as experimental, or even as a frivolity on a par with a nose job. . . . After twenty years of scientific advances, nearly three out of four couples seeking assisted reproduction still go home to an empty crib."[34]

And the author didn't even mention infertility's impact on the marriage relationship—which is substantial. As we will discuss in the next chapter, part of the challenge is that men are like file drawers; women are like balls of yarn.

DISCUSSION QUESTIONS

1. What preconceived ideas did you have about infertility, and how accurate were they?
2. Which, if any, of the above myths and facts surprised you?
3. Which, if any, had you already heard?
4. What did you think when you heard them?
5. What is the most outlandish thing you've heard about infertility?
6. What other myths have people told you?

Chapter 3

Marital Dynamics

She Wants a Baby; He Wants His Wife Back

"Give me children, or I'll die!" (Rachel, Gen. 30:1).

I've told my husband that he should leave me. But since he wouldn't leave me, I said I should die so he could have a better life. Yet somehow we've hung in there.

We had just finished speaking at an infertility symposium and sat down to eat lunch. Moments later, an infertile couple attending the conference joined us. As they began to share their pain, it became apparent that infertility was negatively affecting their marriage. We asked some questions, trying to ascertain how we might help, and their answers were very revealing.

We asked the wife, "When you grieve over your infertility, what is your greatest loss?" She didn't even have to think before answering. "It's the loss of a dream. My heart's desire is to have my husband's child and to raise it with him."

We turned to the husband. "And you?"

He looked at his wife, hesitated, then stroked her arm. His words came gently. "Don't take this wrong, honey, but ..." Then he looked at us. "It's the loss of my wife—she is not the same happy woman I married. I miss her. Infertility is really taking a toll on us."

Such marital stress is a normal result of an abnormal experience. Like most couples, this husband and wife viewed the losses differently.

Not only do men and women tend to respond differently to infertility; they almost never respond the same way at the same time. A study of 269 women and 217 men associated with an infertility clinic found that while men and women often had similar reactions to infertility, the timing and intensity of these reactions differed. Women tended to see more relationship stress arising from infertility than men, and women were also more likely to seek counseling.[1] Often the wife wants to pursue treatment before her husband does, and she's more devastated by the day-to-day disappointments. The husband wants his wife to "stop obsessing" and feels he must be "strong."

As mentioned earlier, throughout this book, we will include quotes, set in italics, from a broad sampling of patients, such as this woman who felt that she and her spouse were worlds apart during infertility:

> *My husband did not understand the loss of self-image that I was feeling, perhaps because men do not define themselves in the same ways that women do. He simply could not relate to what I was going through. Many times his actions and words inadvertently contributed to my loss of self-image.*

His and Hers: We Are So Different!

When infertility occurs, undergoing treatment is often the first real crisis a couple has faced together. And while we hesitate to make generalizations, when it comes to infertility, we have seen that recurring patterns often seem to fall along fairly gender-specific lines.

Men's and women's responses go far beyond the obvious physical differences. Certainly women's reproductive systems are on the "inside" and men's are on the "outside." The testing for men is relatively straightforward (though men often feel uncomfortable about masturbating to produce a semen sample), while testing for women involves regular exploration of the "inner spaces." And women's hormones operate in a complex symphony, whereas men's hormones are relatively simple. Yet try to list other differences, and the picture gets fuzzier.

Researchers once believed that gender-specific social differences were innate—something we were born with. But after further research, they leaned toward attributing these differences to social factors (nurture). Today many researchers suggest it may be some of both, nature and nurture, though it's hard to assess exactly how that works. We don't claim to know whether men's and women's general responses to infertility are due to nature or nurture. We just know that we've observed couples' responses to infertility frequently enough to know that even those husbands and wives most committed to equal social roles respond to infertility with fairly predictable patterns. Many husbands and wives have been shocked to discover how differently they process the experience. And we've seen how helping couples to anticipate and handle their differences helps them to communicate better and to find a place of oneness in their relationship. This ultimately removes some of the marital stress caused by infertility.

Cultural and Background Differences

Ana and her husband, Armando, came from two different continents, two different cultures. In Armando's country of origin, people viewed infertility as a punishment from God. Armando was pursuing higher education in Christian leadership when Ana learned that she had polycystic ovaries. They not only experienced the normal grief that comes from facing infertility; they also felt pressure to achieve a pregnancy so they could pursue career goals. They saw the need to educate people in Armando's country that infertility is *not* a punishment from God, but they knew they would be unable even to gain a hearing without the prerequisite children.

Each person brings background influences to the infertility equation. Most little girls grow up saying, "I want to be a mommy some day." (In health classes, students learn to prevent conception, but rarely does anyone mention infertility. Fertility—even "excess fertility"—is assumed.) When meeting a couple for the first time, people usually ask the husband, "What do you do?" while they ask the wife, "How many children do you have?" Young moms frequently discuss their childbirth experiences; young fathers generally don't. According to one researcher, even women with high-powered careers tend to view their primary role in life as "mommy" before "businesswoman." Traditionally, fertility has been more central to a woman's identity than to a man's.

"The emotions that surround infertility are emotions associated with loss," according to Dan Clements, former board chairman of RESOLVE, a consumer group for infertility patients and providers. "For men who see their primary role in life as working outside the home, the loss related to infertility is the loss of a secondary role: that of being a father. But for women it is the loss of a primary role, that of being a mother."[2] The husband who considers what it might be like to lose the ability to work can appreciate in a new way the depth of his wife's pain. Conversely, a wife can better empathize with her husband's grief by recognizing that her primary loss is much different from his: the loss of a happy, functioning partner.

Consider other influences that may be different for each couple. The husband with male-factor infertility may link his sense of manhood with virility. "Fertility, masculinity and potency are concepts that are often equated," write therapists Ellen Glazer and Susan Cooper. "It is understandable, therefore, that when a man is given a diagnosis of infertility, his identity as a man suffers a real setback. He can easily feel impotent and emasculated. Sometimes men with no prior history of sexual inadequacy or dysfunction become impotent for periods of time after they learn about their infertility problem."[3]

Perhaps the husband's family loves to research genealogy, and now he wonders, "What's the point?" Or maybe the wife had a wonderful childhood, so she grieves that she will never give her parents grand-children. One patient, Barbara, wrote, "I was keenly aware that I could not share with my mother the joys of being a parent. It dawned on me that, although infertility was my experience and my loss, perhaps it was a loss for her as well. The child that my husband and I dreamed of ... would also be an extension of our family—someone's niece or nephew, grandchild, and cousin. This would be the ultimate gift to share with our family: a child."

Differences in How We Process Data

Research suggests that men tend to think in compartments, with one subject at a time having their complete focus; women tend to think more "globally." In a woman's world, nearly everything is connected in some way.[4] Thus, we sometimes liken men to file drawers and women to balls of yarn.

Many wives report that they can talk on the phone, cook dinner, and nod answers to questions all at the same time. Yet if they try talking to their husbands during a TV show—even during the commercials—their words fall on deaf ears. Men often find that their concentration is on what's in their field of vision, and the hearing pathways are not oper-ational in those moments. Thus, we see two different approaches—one focused, one global. Neither is right or wrong, just different.

How might this look for a couple in treatment? For the woman, all roads lead to a baby. The struggle to achieve and maintain a pregnancy has emotional, medical, spiritual, ethical, financial, and relational ram-ifications. So while she's at work, she's thinking about what the doctor said. While she's ordering something on the internet, she clicks over and checks out an infertility website. As she runs errands, she considers her sadness, or while she's at a party, she wonders who might say some-thing insensitive. She might want to have seemingly endless conversa-tions with the man she loves about how she feels, and she'll want to hear how he feels.

Her husband, even if he is grieving deeply, has an "infertility drawer" in the file cabinet. When he opens that drawer, he feels sad. But he can close that drawer and open another and not feel sad. The infer-tility drawer is shut. He might even prefer to keep it shut so he will feel less emotional pain. While it's shut, he can enjoy other facets of life—

friends, sports, jokes. The sight of babies or pregnant women may not affect him. His wife may interpret this as lack of caring. She reasons, "If he were hurting as much as I am, he would notice those things."

The "compartmental" male will work all day without giving much thought to infertility, while the "global" wife goes through her day thinking about virtually nothing else. Only as the infertility lifestyle drags on from months to years does he begin to see that he and his wife probably won't have biological children, and only then does he begin to think more passionately about these issues. But even then, his passion may never appear to match hers. (Of course, these are generalizations. About 20 percent of the time, couples report that this dynamic is reversed, with the wife being more compartmental and the husband more global.)

Longing to "have his happy wife back," the husband typically suggests that she "get her mind off of it." He may even suggest quitting treatment to help her find normalcy again. He is willing to sacrifice even their dreams of a child so she can return to that delightful person he fell in love with. That willingness to sacrifice stems from love. Yet for his grieving wife, the suggestion that they stop treatment comes off as the ultimate act of insensitivity. She may view him as being uncaring or uncommitted to having children. The end result: a husband who's trying to comfort his wife, and a wife who feels abandoned.

Now add the fact that women tend to read more than men. Thus, a woman going through treatment may be able to describe every test, pronounce every medical term, cite clinic-specific success rates, and rattle off the web addresses of everyone who has ever done infertility work. She may be a year or two ahead of her husband in considering adoption. She may find answers to her questions and lay some of her fears to rest as she gathers more information. And her husband may feel out of step with her. As one wife wrote, "For a long time it was just me falling apart and him trying to hold things together. It wasn't until many losses and years later that he started showing signs of falling apart, and by then I had the strength to support him through it."

In such cases, the husband and wife are walking on parallel paths, but they aren't walking side by side. As one wife expressed it, "We have never been on the same page at the same time." Another said, "My husband wondered why I wasn't feeling better; I wondered why he wasn't feeling worse. And the feelings of failure overwhelmed me."

Differences in Communication Styles

The average woman speaks roughly twice as many words as her male counterpart on any given day. According to one linguist, men say three times as many words in public as they do in private, while for women the reverse is true.[5] Not only is her "word count" higher than his, but it's probably at its highest when she's alone with him.

When we poll American women about their five greatest needs, conversation shows up near the top of the list. Nothing that requires using words ever shows up on men's needs lists (unless you count moaning).

Men and women today tend to have different views of the purpose of conversation and different approaches. Men generally report, while women talk to build rapport. Most men talk facts, while most women talk facts *and* feelings.[6] Men actually have fewer fibers connecting the verbal and emotional sides of the brain than do women[7] and use mostly the left side of the brain when listening. Women use both. The findings here don't necessarily mean women are better listeners. Rather, it may mean simply that listening is harder for men.

So here's how it plays out. A wife may ask, "How was your day?" and receive "Fine" as the answer. Her husband intends this to qualify as a satisfactory response and is not trying to avoid her. He has little to report. In one man's words, "I've just lived through this incredibly routine day. Why would I want to relive it by talking about it?"

Yet when a husband asks his wife about *her* day, he may receive more than five thousand words about what traffic was like on her way to work, the meeting she had that morning, and her lunch with a friend. She might even cite the names of the people she called that afternoon and what they said.

By this time, he may be tapping his foot. "Because so much of their own conversation is goal-oriented and functional, men may be hard-pressed to understand much of women's conversation and sit there waiting for them to 'get to the point,'" explains Dr. Elaine Storkey, author of *Origins of Difference*. "For most women, on the other hand, the conversation *is* the point."[8] By taking him along with her on this verbal trip, she is drawing him into her world.

"Many of our disagreements come from equally valid, if different, points of view," say researchers. "What women may regard as intimacy feels suffocating and invasive to men. What many men regard as masculine strength feels isolating and distant to women."[9]

How does this look when infertility is thrown into the mix? An infertile wife's conversation is filled with medical details, hurtful comments made to her, and how she's feeling. She expresses her fears. She wonders aloud what her future will hold. When she asks her husband for the millionth time if they can talk about infertility or adoption, his eyes glaze over. He wonders, "What is left to talk about?"

Generally, women's most frequently expressed complaint about their husbands is that they don't listen, so it should come as no surprise that we see this dynamic emphasized when a couple faces extra stress. (Men's most frequently expressed complaint is that their wives are always trying to change them.)[10]

Some couples have found it helpful to agree ahead of time that they will limit their talk about infertility to twenty to thirty minutes a day. This motivates the wife to focus on what she most wants to communicate, and it assures the husband there will be limits on the amount of time and energy spent focused on infertility.

Most couples already talk too little for building a happy, healthy relationship, so we also recommend allotting time for discussing other issues. Deep communication and verbal intimacy go far beyond infertility information. Such communication needs to be bilateral; that is, the husband must agree to communicate his thoughts and feelings. It's hard to fill twenty minutes with "fine," "weather's fine," "how 'bout that football team?" A wife needs to hear from her husband.

As the husband strives to interact sensitively with his wife, he becomes attuned to the grief triggers for her (pregnant women, babies, that nosy aunt at family gatherings) and responds. He recognizes these situations, confides in her, and shows sensitivity to her hurts. She gets her needs met, and he gets what he wants: a more contented spouse.

Differences in Problem-Solving Approaches

Another difference surfaces in how men and women tend to approach problem solving. Women often respond to situations more immediately and spontaneously than men, finding it difficult to distance themselves from the way they feel. Men tend to more easily detach themselves from emotions and immediate reactions. Also, women often share their problems, looking for commiseration, while men may share only when seeking a solution.

A man whose wife had a stillborn baby was talking with an infertility patient who had just miscarried. He asked how the woman's husband was handling their difficulty, and she answered, "He doesn't seem to grieve much."

"Did you two have a cradle already?"

"Yes."

"What happened to it after your loss?"

The woman thought a moment. "Huh. It used to be in the nursery and then somehow I guess it ended up in the attic."

The man nodded. "I guarantee your husband hauled it up there while you weren't around so you wouldn't have to watch."

Tears suddenly filled her eyes.

"I carried our cradle up into the attic after we lost our baby, too. Trust me—he's grieving. He's just doing it differently than you."

It's important to look beyond a spouse's actions to see how he or she may be communicating love and loss, rather than assuming "I'm the only one doing the grief work here." Husbands and wives often assume they'll mourn the exact same way, and this misconception can polarize them. It helps to ask for what you need rather than hoping your spouse will guess and get it right.

My husband started going with me to medical appointments. Not only did that make me feel loved; it also gave us an extra set of ears to hear what the doctor said.

I have to be specific about my needs, like asking my husband to hold me each month when my period again begins. Also, a therapist advised us that we can try working for a cause, some joint project that is larger than ourselves.

It was a big deal to me when my husband began referring to infertility as "our" problem instead of "my" problem. I've heard some men don't realize that they're not going to be biological fathers until they're filling out adoption papers.

A wife can't read her husband's mind, and he can't read hers. And he usually can't take hints; that skill was never wired into the male hard drive. So spare yourselves plenty of hurt. If you need a hug without it leading anywhere, say so. Just be sure not to neglect intimacy at other times of the cycle (more on this later).

Other Differences

Researchers who work specifically with infertile couples have found further expressions of gender-specific responses.

1. *Wives* may view pregnancy and childbirth as a strong yearning, perhaps even a biological need; *husbands* may view it more in terms of reproducing their genes and passing along their line.
2. *Women* tend to demonstrate more outward expressions of emotion; *men* tend to be more detached. This may be exacerbated by his sense of not being part of the treatment, as even when a male factor is involved, it is usually the woman who undergoes most of the treatment.
3. Studies suggest that when infertility is first discovered, *women* react in a more emotionally devastated manner; *men* seem to have a more optimistic outlook on treatment possibilities. These

same studies suggest, however, that as treatment becomes prolonged, both parties may become dispirited.

4. *Women* may find relief by expressing emotions and telling oth-
    ers what is happening; *men* typically value their privacy, partic-
    ularly if a male factor is involved. This may be why studies have
    shown that marriages of infertile couples are more at risk when
    a male factor is involved.[11]

5. Fifty percent of infertile *women* who responded to one study said
    their infertility was the greatest burden they had ever had to bear;
    only 15 percent of the *men* responding said the same thing.[12]

6. A psychologist found in a poll of *husbands* that on a scale of zero
    to ten, with ten being "in control," the average man felt he rated
    a six in assessing his own emotional response to fertility treat-
    ment. When asked the question, "To what degree did you feel
    your *wife* was emotionally in control during your infertility
    experience?" the average man answered three.[13]

Being at such different places along the path can be especially serious when you feel you no longer identify with the other's feelings. In
the most serious cases, couples stop communicating altogether. A husband who just wants his life to "get back to normal" may move from
wanting to help his wife stop the pain to outright blaming her that they
no longer enjoy activities together. It's important to understand each
other's reactions as reasonable behavior and to take steps to handle in
a healthy way the differences we've described.

De-Stressing the Marriage

Marriage experts have concluded that none of these differences—
personality, background, gender—cause the greatest marital problems.
The most serious problems are caused by how we *handle* our differences.
As researchers in one major study concluded, "The things we *can* control cause the most damage."[14] In other words, how we choose to
respond is the crucial factor. Part of handling infertility well is understanding and accepting that the typical patterns couples experience are
normal.

People often think that the key to a happy marriage is finding the
right person, but it's more about being or becoming the right person.
After hearing this idea at one of our conferences, a husband and wife
told us, "We had been thinking maybe we weren't meant for each other.
But now we see that the stress would be hard on any couple and we
need to strengthen our relationship."

A therapist who deals primarily with infertility patients insists that in
a healthy marriage, a couple undergoing treatment should expect to

receive only about 30 percent of their support from each other. God designed us for community, and most of our relational needs are met in a network of support that extends beyond the marriage. "For generations women have gathered over coffee or quilts; men have bonded at work and in taverns," wrote researchers Aaron Kipnis and Elizabeth Herron. "But in our modern society, most heterosexuals believe that a member of the opposite sex is supposed to fulfill all their emotional and social needs."[15]

Gail and I are infertility phone buddies. We met in an ultrasound waiting room, where, with our bladders painfully full, we wincingly exchanged our phone numbers and immediately embarked on an intimate new friendship because those closest to us no longer comprehend us.

Expecting too much from one's marriage puts stress on it, so couples need to look for additional sources of support. Informal patient-led support groups can be terrific sources of information and encouragement. Prayer groups are great too. If people say the wrong thing, gently help them see how their words hurt you. Get on the internet and connect with an "infertility buddy." (We've listed some websites in the Resources section at the back of the book.) One writer attributes such groups with saving her marriage:

The several support groups to which I belong get the most credit for helping me face infertility. I needed someone to tell me what I felt was normal. I believed I was crazy because that's what the people around me told me. Before I got involved with online groups, I went to grief counseling, which led to a couples' RESOLVE group. These were the beginning of my recovery.[16]

According to some research, infertile couples are no more prone to marital breakup than are any other couples. In fact, many couples find that they are capable of supporting one another and working through their personal crisis in such a way that, if anything, their relationships are stronger than ever.[17]

After three years of treatment, Suzanne felt frustrated with her husband because he rarely went with her to support groups or information meetings. But one afternoon she saw him through new eyes: "The day my doctor told me I might never have children, I sobbed. Then I called my husband and told him. His voice was so gentle. He said, 'That's too bad ...' I asked him how he felt, and he said he was sorry about it, but he was okay. I said, 'Don't you feel ripped off?' He said, 'Honey, it's out of our control. Neither of us knew or could have known that there was a problem. The Lord is in control.' I argued, 'But you married me thinking we'd have kids, and now I'm keeping you from our dream. You'd probably be better off finding someone fertile.' He said, 'What? No way! If I had the choice between somebody else with kids or you with no kids, I'd choose you.'"

Suzanne concluded, "I knew he loved me, but it took infertility for me to see just how much."

Infertile couples often emerge from the experience saying, as one patient expressed, "I feel like we've lived the worst; we can survive anything now." Her friend echoed her sentiment: "I know now that come hell or high water, we'll be together and we'll get through."

DISCUSSION QUESTIONS

1. How much time do you as a couple spend talking about infertility? About other topics?
2. Would you say you and your spouse are able to have fun despite infertility, or is all the joy gone?
3. What memories are the two of you building now?
4. Do you feel you're deepening the friendship part of your marriage? Why or why not?
5. Do you ever laugh together? What makes you laugh?
6. Would you say you're kind to each other? How can you improve in this area?
7. Check out a website that has stress questionnaires with feedback (such as stressdiagnosis.com or cliving.org). Take the test and discuss your results with your spouse (or the members of your support group). What can you do to decrease the stress in your lives?
8. What is the financial impact of your treatment plan? Are you going into debt? If so, are you both comfortable with the level of debt incurred? Is the money question putting additional stress on your marriage?
9. Take twenty to thirty minutes to talk about what you enjoy doing, both individually and together.
10. Ask each other the following: What activity would you like to do that's unrelated to infertility? A ball game? A movie? A quiet night of conversation without talking about infertility?
11. Make separate lists of five topics unrelated to infertility that you'd enjoy discussing (such as your favorite vacation) and talk through them, alternating with one from each of your lists.

Chapter 4

EMOTIONAL DYNAMICS

The emotional pain associated with infertility is excruciating. There's the loneliness, the lack of control, stressed relationships, sleep problems, sexual dysfunction, waiting to hear from the doctor's office, delayed decisions, career stagnation, withdrawal from family and friends, debt, insurance hassles, unending and invasive exams, medically induced emotional swings, daily trips to the lab ... punctuated each month with "I started my period."

In the past three decades, researchers have made great strides in the treatment of infertility. They've figured out how to freeze and thaw eggs, how to transfer embryos, how to inject a single sperm into an egg, using a miniature pipette. Yet all of that is the relatively simple part. The more difficult part is mending the broken hearts.

"The literature has tended to show that women regard infertility as the most disastrous thing that's ever happened to them," says a psychiatrist who specializes in treating infertility patients. One study from Harvard Medical School found that women with infertility had levels of emotional distress equal to those of patients with cancer or heart disease. For every failed attempt to conceive, couples experience grief for what could have been. As this is repeated month after month, sometimes for years, it becomes chronic grief.[1]

One man, the father of two biological children, teaching a church class on ethics said, "These infertile couples are totally obsessing over having kids. There are so many needy children already out there. This high-tech stuff that circumvents conception is a futile attempt at 'playing God.' It just demonstrates how people are too stuck on genetics." The infertile couples in the class sat and reeled from the impact of his words. Could he be right? It seemed logical enough—simple supply and demand. Yet they found it hard to let go of the notion of genetic immortality, of the desire to conceive a child together, of the desire to experience pregnancy together. Did that mean they were stuck on genetics? Did their intense emotional response mean they were obsessing?

Consider the story of Hannah, found in 1 Samuel 1. (We'll explore her story in-depth in chapter 6.) Hannah was a godly woman who was unable to conceive. She cried, lost her appetite, saw things differently from how her husband did, bargained with God, and prayed. Observing her distress, the priest at the temple thought she was drunk, but the writer of the biblical narrative presents her as a woman of faith who reacted intensely to her situation.

We see from Hannah's story that the feelings of loss associated with infertility are normal, and the drive to have biological children is healthy and natural. Yet frequently patients describing their emotions exclaim, "I feel like I'm going crazy!"

Infertility is the gradual death of a dream. Rather than following a set list of stages, a patient tends to spiral through them and bounce back and forth, with no clear beginning and ending to the stages. Also unique to infertility is the fact that at certain times of the month, the patient often has hope that "this will be the month." That hope can turn to despair when the period starts and the cycle begins again.

Mary, an infertility patient, observed, "The unsuccessful attempt to have a child is really a loss within a loss. An infertility patient experiences a monthly cycle of hope and despair that falls within the much longer grieving process." Mary was working on an advanced degree while she and her husband were in treatment. As part of her education, she took a psychology class, in which students discussed the emotions associated with facing a terminal illness. She noticed that infertility patients experience many of the same emotions.

Grieving the Phantom Child
Denial

I hated the way medical tests were cutting into my work. I still didn't want to believe there was anything wrong.

We've been trying for two years to have a baby. But it's not that I'm infertile—I'm just having trouble getting pregnant. I was asked to edit a newsletter for fertility patients, but I declined. My reason: I was going to be pregnant soon.

The doctor says we're infertile. What does he know?

I thought about talking to a friend who has also had trouble having a baby. Yet that seems extreme. She's infertile; I'm just taking a long time to get pregnant. There's no point even seeing a doctor yet. It's been only a year since we started trying.

I can't believe this is real. Nothing prepared me for this. Nothing!

Anger

I was and am angry! Despite bad things happening to good people and the lessons we learn from Job, I've told God I am not Job. He seems to have answered back with, "Maybe you should be." I've contemplated many horrible things I never thought I'd contemplate.

When I first heard that infertility patients were often angry, I thought they lacked spiritual maturity—God doesn't owe anybody a child. Now I see that I felt that way only because I had not yet been broken as badly as they had. Well, now I have . . . and I'm angry!

I'm upset about what isn't and what won't be . . . angry at feeling so alone with no support and no money to pay for a counselor.

Five years after I miscarried, my sister—after weeks of angst—called to tell me that she was pregnant again. I screamed at heaven, "You cannot ask me to do this again!"

Everything makes me angry, and I know much of my anger is misdirected. I'm angry at my body, my partner, my family, my medical team, and my insurance company.

Bargaining

I've given up Pepsi to rid my body of caffeine. Hopefully God will see how serious I am about having a baby.

I keep trying to think of what thing I can do—give up alcohol, quit going to school, sell my car, move into a hut—that will show I'm worthy. I've tried a lot of stuff, but nothing seems to work.

I don't sew or cook very well, but one day I found myself entering a fabric store. I began examining bolts of material. Somewhere inside, I believed that if I learned to sew—became more domestic—then I might deserve to have a baby.

Depression

Infertility makes me feel like my pain is as bottomless as the Grand Canyon, my barrenness like Death Valley. I want to hide with my head under the covers.

I avoid people, especially the mall—especially at Christmas! I've pulled back in friendships with pregnant women and moms.

I have trouble concentrating at work. I feel guilty that my medical stuff is keeping my wife from being what she's always dreamed—a mommy.

Often depression is accompanied by a deep crisis of faith.

I didn't feel it at first, but after several losses and failed adoptions, I started to believe God thought I didn't deserve to be a parent. It didn't make sense to me that he would single me out.

I never felt that anyone in the church was sympathetic to my situation.

I was close to losing my faith. I felt God had abandoned and betrayed me. He didn't protect me from loss when I prayed and pleaded for him to do so. So many bad things could not be happening to me if God were watching out for me.

I wondered if I'd really made some bad mistakes and this was my punishment. I started thinking I must be a bad person.

I found it painful to attend services, and I stopped going to church for a long time. It was difficult to witness the baptisms, the families, the pregnant congregants. It was difficult to hear insensitive comments and have people tell me that my losses were "God's plan." I felt like no one understood how I felt, and worse yet, I felt that they were judging me.

Mourning

Last year on Mother's Day, I was listening to a radio interview of a Pulitzer Prize winner and her mother, and I didn't like the way they described their relationship. I thought about how I'd want a relationship with my own daughter to be different and what values I'd instill in her. Suddenly the realization that I'd never have that chance overwhelmed me. I sobbed for a long time.

My heart was broken and my arms ached with emptiness. Now with our dreams of having children lying shredded at my feet, the anguish of my soul again sought expression in tears and prayers, but it seemed there was no answer. I wanted to sit in sackcloth and ashes, wailing until I lost consciousness.

I shut myself in my home office and cried for hours. Not long after that, someone put a guilt trip on me for not adopting a four-year-old. I don't need that. It's bad enough to consider never giving birth. But to miss the first smile, the first tooth, getting to name my own child. Too many losses. I'm facing that I'll never give birth, and it hurts a lot.

Each time my period comes it's like a little death. I cry, or worse, feel numb.

Acceptance

I think that before you are ready to stop treatment it feels like quitting. Once I've made peace with infertility, it feels like moving on.

We planted a tree in our yard and dedicated it to all the children that didn't get to be with us in this life. I thought it would be hard to walk away from infertility treatments, but that simple little act gave me a concrete ending and made the transition for me.

At one time I said we would never adopt—that option looked awful to me. Now I'm actually starting to get excited when I think about it.

I made one last appointment with the endocrinologist. He told me about an experimental therapy I could try, but it was still in trials, so I might get a placebo, and it would require the discipline of a football player in training. No thanks.

Suggestions for Managing the Emotional Crisis

There is no "right" way to grieve, and a patient does not necessarily experience each of the emotions just described. But if you've felt this wide range of emotions, you're not crazy and you're not alone. Here are some suggestions for helping you manage the emotions associated with infertility.

Know that emotions are part of God's design. Infertility causes pain, hurt, loss, grief. And it's okay to feel intense negative emotions; it's just not okay to let them lead us into sin. (Ephesians 4:26 tells us, "In your anger do not sin.") Jesus wept at Lazarus' tomb, even though he knew he could raise him from the dead. Emotions do not necessarily represent a lack of faith.

Worship. In the Scriptures, we read about Job's response when he learned he had lost all his material possessions and then all of his children: "At this, Job got up and tore his robe and shaved his head. Then he fell to the ground in worship and said: 'Naked I came from my mother's womb, and naked I will depart. The LORD gave and the LORD has taken away; may the name of the LORD be praised.' In all this, Job did not sin by charging God with wrongdoing" (Job 1:20–22).

Months after my pregnancy loss, I've found it harder to worship as the pain wears on, but I still make it a priority. Initially when the shock hit, all I could do was tell God, "I don't understand what You're doing, but You're God and I'm not ..." Singing my heart out through my tears reminds me that there's more to this life than what's in front of me in the moment. I keep my CD player stocked with praise and worship music.

If you have a relationship with God, you have a definite advantage over someone who walks alone. In addition, your church community is a logical place to seek out the comfort of those who should be in a good position to help you. You might have to explain to a few friends what you need from them, but find a prayer group or a small discussion group with whom you can bare your soul. Jesus, who never married and who had no children, spoke often of the spiritual family bond being stronger than that of the biological family.

Work to keep your marriage strong. You can find a variety of ways to strengthen your marriage relationship without spending much money. Visit museums together, rent videos, drive to the beach, go camping, read to each other. One couple said, "Even the best relationships can learn something new. So we've decided to read and discuss at least one book each year about marriage."[2]

Decide to live "one day at a time." "Many mornings I would get up and tell myself, 'Okay, I know I'm obviously not going to become a mom today. I'm not even going to conceive today. Maybe someday . . . but not today,'" Marissa wrote after three years of unexplained infertility. "So I'd ask myself, 'How can I make the best of where I am now— to enjoy life to the fullest in other areas while I wait?'" Marissa ended up getting a master's degree that made it possible to work from home when she later adopted.

Jesus taught his disciples, "Do not worry about tomorrow, for tomorrow will worry about itself. Each day has enough trouble of its own" (Matt. 6:34).

Temporarily avoid situations that are too painful. Allow yourself a healthy avoidance of some situations that, for now, evoke emotions you can't resolve. It may be the Thanksgiving dinner with eight nieces and nephews, or perhaps it's the baby shower for a coworker. These situations do more than remind you of your losses; they can also make you self-conscious that you are ruining the event for others. During some seasons, the most spiritual thing you can do for your overall health and spiritual well-being is to absent yourself from large gatherings.

Talk to others. Hurting people usually find relief through talking about their problems with an empathic listener. Yet verbally processing the loss may bring more relief for the wife than for the husband. After baring his soul, a man may express, "Now I feel worse." Nevertheless, men need to find ways to express their feelings. As one man noted, "When I try to keep the 'grief drawer' shut for long enough, if I refuse to open it, eventually it kicks itself open." So find an "infertility buddy," a mentor, a fellowship group, an infertility support group, and/or a good counselor who supports your faith worldview.

"My church doesn't have an infertility support group," Susan wrote, "but I attend one at another church. It has been my lifeline." Some research suggests that patients who attend support groups sometimes end up having higher pregnancy rates than those who don't.[3] Though some connect this with an alleviation of stress, there may be additional factors. For example, by exchanging information with others who are in treatment, patients quickly learn which doctors specialize in what sort of treatments, and they hear about new treatment options and available resources. They may also find that their friends hold them to their decisions to be more active in managing their medical care.

In one study, couples who attended an average of three out of five group therapy sessions during an in vitro fertilization (IVF) cycle demonstrated that the support did help in tangible ways. The women reported significantly less anxiety and depression than the control group did. The men became more optimistic, unlike men who did not participate in the group sessions. The researchers noted, "It would appear from these data that both men and women benefit from group participation, albeit in different ways."[4]

Find creative outlets for expressing grief. Journaling, writing poetry, or painting may provide effective outlets for expressing one's grief. A couple who lost their only son told of spending Thanksgiving serving the homeless to take their minds off their son's empty place at the dinner table.

Couples often find that it helps to create their own unique, lame brand of humor. Gary and I chose to "redefine Webster" during a particularly frustrating week. Here's a sampling of our new definitions:

Family reunion: An opportunity to hear all the existing myths about infertility.

Time (two syllables, as in, "Honey, it's ti-ime"): Rare event around which the rest of life orbits.

BBT Chart (Basal Body Temperature Chart): Record of daily mood swings as determined by basal thermometer.

Take care of yourself. The endorphins released during a workout or lovemaking (or from laughter, chocolate, and chili peppers—not all at the same time) act as natural mood elevators. Exercise helps to create a sense of well-being. In addition, couples need to express sexual intimacy at times other than fertile days.

Our bodies need adequate rest and an abundance of healthful foods. Too much or too little body fat, especially for women, may impact fertility.[5] Smoking, excessive use of alcohol, and caffeine have also been shown to have an adverse effect on fertility. Rest, exercise, good nutrition, and stress avoidance work to help patients combat anxiety.

Read. Some people feel discouraged after reading medical literature, but others find comfort in being armed with the latest and best information available. In most libraries, you can find a database with current medical data, which is better than reading popular magazines, which run a year or two behind the latest data. Some patients feel better after reading through counseling materials about the emotions associated with their specific losses, finding validation in the stories of others who have felt the same way. Many patients park themselves on the internet. Sites such as www.inciid.org and www.conceivingcon cepts.org provide a wealth of information. But be careful. We checked out a bogus website that cited an outlandish success rate for using massage to treat fibroids. So read with a healthy skepticism! (Note: One spouse may prefer to avoid doing research, and it is unnecessary for both to share the same degree of interest here.)

Find a medical team you can trust. In most cases, the staff at a clinic is as important as the physician. You'll never get perfection, but you should be able to find competence and compassion. Having a good rapport with your medical team can greatly reduce the stress you experience. (More on finding a medical team in chapter 11.)

Know that healing takes time—usually longer than you expect and much longer than most North Americans are used to allowing. It has been said that "time heals all wounds." Yet time itself does not heal. Time and lamenting and praying and struggling and continuing to move forward should bring healing. Having a good listener who loves you well expedites the process.

And healing doesn't have to mean forgetting. Some losses we wouldn't *want* to forget. A mother who lost a pregnancy after infertility said that though she appreciated being able to finally return to "functioning," she wouldn't want to heal completely if it meant she had to forget the human life that she and her husband had conceived.

Delay making major decisions if you've just been through a failed IVF cycle, a pregnancy loss, or even a week in which eight friends have announced their pregnancies. Grief can impair good judgment and can make you feel indecisive. When pain and grief are severe, just deciding what to eat for dinner can feel like a major chore.

***Recognize that holidays and anniversaries can be especially diffi-
cult.*** Levels of depression in the general population tend to increase
during the holidays. In a season during which everyone else in the
world seems to be celebrating, a season when we hear, "Christmas is for
the children," the infertile couple can feel like they're outside, looking
in the window at all the festivities. One patient wrote, "In the holy season, I identify less with the Magi and more with those whose children
Herod killed: 'In Rama there was a voice heard, lamentation, and weeping, and great mourning, Rachel weeping for her children, and would
not be comforted, because they are no more'" (Matt. 2:18 KJV).

Seek to give something back. Look for ways to use your pain as a
bridge to help others who also hurt. One woman wrote, "I've been
involved in pregnancy loss support for a long time, and I have created
plaques in memory of lost children. The parents can display them
prominently or just keep them in a safe place." Through comforting others, this woman experiences comfort herself.

Pray and cry out to God. In the midst of my pain, I (Sandi) found
myself continually drawn to the Psalms after my pregnancy losses. New
phrases such as "How long, O LORD?" (6:3) and "My God, my God, why
have you forsaken me?" (22:1) began to fill my prayers. While echoing
these spiritual gripes, I discovered, to my surprise, that the lament is
the most common form of psalm in the Bible. Perhaps if we followed
inspired examples of legitimized whining—if we spent more time fuss-
ing to God than to therapists—we'd write fewer checks for couch time.
It's also helpful to write out our prayers. Here's a psalm of lament I
wrote after miscarrying repeatedly.

> *O Lord, not again.*
> *How could you allow this again?*
> *Once more the doctor has said our baby's gone, and I feel pain deeper
> than my own soul.*
> *Our friends say, "Maybe you can have another," but why would you
> let me conceive this one if it wasn't going to live?*
> *I want this child, Lord! How long must we keep going through this
> endless cycle of hope and despair? It feels so cruel.*
> *I hate it and I don't understand it, but I have nowhere to go but to You.*
> *Please help me to trust You.*

Writing and praying my own laments as I experienced multiple
losses helped me honestly express my grief to God. Before Dr. Bill
directed me to the psalms of lament, I had thought it wrong to ask why
this had happened to us or to suggest I might feel any displeasure about

God's ways. Afterward, with new courage to express the pain I felt, I found a deeper respect for the Lord's greatness, amazed that he not only allows us to talk to him this way, but he has even provided in Scripture some examples of how to do so.

Put first things first. Cynthia had been in treatment for several years with no success. "I reached a point where I had to make a choice," she said. "I was working and ministering on the side. I had to decide either to quit teaching the Bible and take a second job to pay for adoption, or to keep using my gifts to serve the Lord. For me, it was an issue of faith. When I was trying to make that decision, I kept thinking about Jesus' exhortation to 'Seek first His kingdom and His righteousness, and all these things [food, clothing] will be added to you' (Matt. 6:33 NASB). Five years later when we were on the verge of adopting, an attorney offered to do our finalization for free. That was a huge confirmation for me. I'm not saying that putting God first means everybody's dreams get fulfilled; it's not a bargaining chip. I simply mean that abundant life comes from the inner life and spiritual priorities, not the outward circumstances and temporal world. Keeping that in perspective has helped us live with no regrets."

Another couple, Thomas and Rebecca, chose to use the freedom currently offered by their childless status to do weeklong overseas mission trips sponsored by their church and a mission board. The good they are able to do helps them see good coming out of their loss in the short term.

Some of these suggestions may sound hard, maybe even annoying, for where you are at this point in the struggle. The fact is, infertility is excruciating; nothing totally takes away the pain. And sadly, you may find that just about the time you're finding a bit of an even keel emotionally, settling into a place of spiritual stability, someone else comes along and dumps peroxide deep into your wound. So how do you help those around you learn to provide support rather than making it worse? Read on.

DISCUSSION QUESTIONS

1. Proverbs 13:12 tells us that "hope deferred makes the heart sick." On a scale of one to ten, how heartsick do you feel? Have your spouse rate himself or herself. What did you predict your spouse would say?

2. As you look back through this chapter, what quotes could have been yours? Why? Did you disagree with any of the thoughts expressed in these quotes? If so, why?

3. How much do you and your spouse research and read about infertility? Or do you prefer to "rock along with the doc"? Is a difference in your approaches ever a source of tension?

4. Which emotion(s) best describes where you are now? Which best describes where your spouse is? Do you ever feel stuck at one place?

5. How has going through infertility impacted your worship experience?

6. Are you tempted to place having a child above your relationship with God? Above your relationship with each other? Which of these receives most of your time and/or energy?

7. Look up the psalms of lament in the Bible. (For a list of lament psalms and their texts, go to www.lament.org.) Do any of them express how you feel?

8. Write your own lament. Tell God what hurts and what you want him to do about it. Try to end your lament with an expression of trust.

Chapter 5

HANDLING
WELL-INTENTIONED ADVICE

Advice is a dangerous gift, even from the wise to the wise, and all courses may run ill.

—Gildor to Frodo, *The Lord of the Rings*

Suzanne had been through two years of intensive medical treatment for infertility. A woman whose friends described her as "reserved," Suzanne had never talked about her emotional pain with anyone besides her husband and a close friend. At the urging of that friend, Suzanne determined to be more open with others about what she was going through rather than closing herself off from support. The following week when she sat with her prayer group and the leader asked, "Does anyone have something they'd like to have us pray about?" Suzanne took a deep breath.

"Uh ... yeah, I do."

All eyes were on her.

"I would like prayer for my husband and me. We've been seeking medical treatment for ..."—she paused, having never actually said the word in public—"uh ... for infertility."

At first the group sat in silence. Then one of the women broke the ice. "Maybe you just need to relax."

Another added, "I know someone who tried for thirteen years and finally got pregnant."

If there's one universal truth about infertility, it's that people often say the wrong thing! Back in Rachel and Leah's time, the advice of the day was, "Get some mandrakes." Hannah must have heard, "Of *course* you're infertile; you've hacked off the fertility god by worshiping only the Lord. Bow down to Baal." Today infertile people hear, "Just relax."

Years ago we noticed that whenever we're in a room full of quiet infertility patients (which is about as rare as a happy infertility patient on Mother's Day), the quickest way to get conversation going is simply to ask, "Has anyone ever said anything insensitive to you about your infertility?" Everyone stares, as if to say, "Duh." Then after that momentary pause, they stumble over each other vying to be the first to tell their horror stories, one-upping each other with, "You think that's bad? Wait'll you hear what my mother-in-law said . . ." Here's a sampling of the sad stories we hear:

> People tell me stuff like, "It's probably for the best—maybe if you got pregnant something would be wrong with the baby," or, "Maybe God's trying to tell you that you'd be bad parents," or my favorite, "Infertility is a curse from God. What did you do wrong?"

> When my sister conceived, I gave family members a book about infertility to help them understand. One responded by saying that I just didn't know how to be happy for anyone else.

> After my pregnancy loss, a friend's mom said, "You must forget it!" I told her I would never forget my first baby. Then she was offended. After that I refrained from mentioning my loss to people who might not understand.

> My husband sat down a few weeks ago and wrote his family a letter telling them if all they could do was say hateful, hurtful words, we would avoid them.

> When I replay scenes in my head, I think of so many things I wish I had said. But it never prepares me for the next insensitive comment. Sometimes I get mad at myself for letting people say the wrong things without setting them straight. But if I try to confront, I might break down, and that would be even worse.

> My favorite is the person who says, "Gee, my husband just looks at me and I get pregnant." I want to say, "Good for you. Now shut your mouth. Like an infertile person would give a rip about how fertile you are."

An old Baptist proverb says, "There is no situation so bad that a little guilt can't make it worse." Some advice-givers are simply rude. Others intend to help but are misguided. They may feel a pressing need to say something—something important, meaningful, and profound. They search their brains to come up with ten words that will change our lives, words that will bring a miraculous solution to the problem. Yet in the absence of true answers or fixes, their "deep and profound words" come out trite and clichéd. Words intended as advice come off as remarkably insensitive and often guilt producing. "The deepest feeling always shows itself in silence; not in silence, but restraint," wrote poet Marianne Moore more than a century ago. Her words still ring true today.

Most of the wrong things people say fall into several broad categories.

The Many Ways of Saying the Wrong Thing

The Problem Solver

"I was infertile too, but when I finally really prayed about it, I conceived."

"Just relax."

"Take a vacation."

"Change doctors."

To the infertile person, suggestions of a basic "fix" feel like blame-the-patient solutions. Problem-solving advice suggests that if only the couple would follow some simple course of action, they'd find a solution. One patient whose husband was sterile due to a congenital abnormality was told, "You just need to pray about it." In response she asked, "Really? You think if I pray, my husband might grow a testicle?"

The Rude Remark

"Want me to show your wife how it's done?"

"You must be doing it wrong!"

"How long have you been married—and you don't have any children yet? Don't you like children?"

Some people are flat clueless. Others are downright rude. In response to the crass person, the only appropriate reply is silence or a bewildered "Why would you *say* something like that?" Some remarks are lame attempts at humor, often spun to suggest that the couple lack knowledge—if only they had more education, they would conceive. Infertile couples know more about LH, FSH, HCG, hysterosalpingograms, and laparoscopies than the fertile nonmedical person would ever want to know.

The "Cheer Up" Remark

"Want kids? Borrow mine for the weekend."

"Be glad you'll never have to deal with having a teenager."

"At least you're having fun trying!"

"Kids are so much work! Enjoy the time you have without them."

"At least . . ."

Often would-be comforters try to cheer those who hurt by mini-mizing their pain. They do so by suggesting that the couple "look at the bright side" to see that "it's not so bad." Such words bring to mind a proverb: "Like one who takes away a garment on a cold day, or like vinegar poured on soda, is one who sings songs to a heavy heart (Prov. 25:20).

> *This kind of "comfort" really backfires. Proverbs says, "He who is full loathes honey, but to the hungry even what is bitter tastes sweet" (Prov. 27:7). When you're starving for something, even the bad parts can seem good. When someone says that I shouldn't feel bad about being infer-tile because having kids is hard, I want to say, "So if someone came and took your children and you never saw them again, you'd be happier?" Of course they don't mean that, but that is how it sounds!*

Another "encouraging statement" gets delivered at baby showers: "Your time will come." First, there is no guarantee that it will. Second, an infertile person sitting at a shower is probably trying to enter into the joy of the one being honored. If attention gets focused on the infer-tile woman's difficulties, she can feel that she is taking away from the unbridled joy of her friend, thus making the infertile woman even more self-conscious. So she may avoid baby showers altogether.

Invalid Validation

"I know exactly how you feel . . ."
Sometimes just when you think you're going to get a little empathy, you find out you've only been set up for a letdown.

> *I shared about my infertility with a friend, and she answered with, "Oh yeah, I know exactly how you feel. It was like that for me when I had postpartum depression."*

> *When I lost a pregnancy, someone told me, "I know just how you feel. When my pet died, I felt like I'd lost a family member."*

No one knows exactly how it feels to walk in another's shoes. Even if someone has been through a similar situation, no two circumstances are exactly the same.

Spiritual Platitudes

"Just trust God."
"Maybe God is trying to . . ."
"What did you do that he's punishing you?"
"It'll all work out in his time."

Of all the advice and unhelpful statements, the most painful are often spiritual statements that suggest grief is either a result of sin or an unholy response to loss.

A friend who used to be infertile told me I shouldn't cry about not having a child because my tears mean I lack faith.

My husband and I are Christians. His family believes that by using ARTs [advanced reproductive technologies] or having surgeries to reduce pain from endometriosis, I am "wielding the hand of God" for my own desires. We've been told, "It'll happen for you! Relax. Adopt. Take a vacation. Don't try so hard." Now they view my apparent barrenness as a judgment from God. My father-in-law said we must not deserve children (as if anyone does). After my pelvic pain got so bad that I had to take narcotic pain medicine, his father said I'm not a mother because I poison my womb. We aren't sinless, but time has taught us that our infertility is not a divine punishment.

A pastor told us, "The most significant thing I learned through my grief was that the high-sounding, though true, theological axioms sound so trite and are immensely irritating. Either God brings those thoughts to your mind with his comfort or they seem of little help."

In the book of Job, we read about a man who, having lost his entire family and everything he owned, lay in agony. His friends came and sat silently with him for a week. Not bad, actually; we don't know too many people who can be silent for an entire week in the face of another's pain. But then they went and opened their mouths. Job's suffering didn't fit their idea of how a just God works. They expected to see clear cause-and-effect relationships in this life; righteous people must prosper, evil people must not. So these "friends" increased Job's suffering by pouring forth their self-proclaimed insight about how God must be punishing him. And it seems that ol' Job grew tired of hearing his "friends" blame the victim. So he mustered up a response: "How you have helped the powerless! How you have saved the arm that is feeble! What advice you have offered to one without wisdom! And what great insight you have displayed! Who has helped you utter these words? And whose spirit spoke from your mouth?" (Job 26:2–4). Can't you just hear his sarcasm?

In our culture, we are often taught to "see the glass as half full," "smile and have a positive attitude," and "keep a stiff upper lip." Yet in the ancient Near East, the picture was much different. "It is better to go to a house of mourning than to go to a house of feasting," we are told, "for death is the destiny of every man; the living should take this to heart" (Eccl. 7:2).

Tears are an appropriate, divinely designed response to intense grief. David, a man after God's own heart, wrote, "In my distress I called to the LORD ... my cry came to his ears" (2 Sam. 22:7). The Psalms are filled with laments showing how the righteous offered their mourning to God. Of the Lord himself we read, "During the days of Jesus' life on earth, he offered up prayers and petitions with loud cries and tears to the one who could save him from death" (Heb. 5:7).

While there may be grains of truth in some of the spiritual statements, sadly they are often used to minimize pain. Those who want infertility patients to consider the spiritual side of their dilemma would do better by asking, "How is this affecting your relationship with God? Does he feel distant, uncaring, unworthy of trust?" They might also consider the apostle Paul's admonition, not to cheer up or preach to those in pain, but to "weep with those who weep" (Rom. 12:15 NASB).

Those who take the time to listen often find that the very people others are labeling as "unspiritual" have, in fact, gained some important insight through their difficulties:

> I wonder where my friends have gone and who I've grown to be. Many of my friends have left me. And I've started to acknowledge it was my own doing. I pushed them away because they had kids and it hurt too much to hear their complaining about the parenting life. As for the person I've grown to be, I've been able to learn a lot about myself. My mind has gotten stronger and my heart bigger. I'm learning to channel my energy into important things like the coming of Christ rather than the new outfit my mother-in-law bought for her granddaughter.

When someone having a great day says, "Trust God," to someone in pain, it sounds like a heartless accusation. It also robs the suffering believer of the opportunity to testify about God's grace. It's the comforter's job to weep; it's the hurting person's job, when he or she is ready, to tell others about God's sufficiency. Too often it happens the other way around. Would-be comforters leave people weeping after "bearing witness" to them that God is sufficient.

The Suffering Olympics

An infertility expert speaking about the doctor-patient relationship shook his head over the stress he sees in infertility patients. Then he pointed down the hall to the cancer ward. "I wish my patients could go look at the people down there. That's the really hard stuff. Maybe it would put their problems into perspective." By the time he'd finished, it was clear that he thought his infertility patients were overreacting. Having not been in their shoes, he was oblivious to how excruciating infertility can be, and he assumed it didn't rank with other forms of pain. Unfortunately, though he spent his life working with infertile people, this doctor was unaware that the depression and anxiety experienced by infertile women are often equivalent to that in women suffering from a terminal illness.

Some patients who have been through both cancer and infertility have said that, for them, infertility was the more difficult of the two. One infertile cancer survivor explains: "I never thought I was going to die of cancer—only that I'd have to endure surgery and radiation. That was short-term. But for me, infertility is long-term—for a lifetime. The prospect of never having children has been worse for me than the diagnosis of cancer."

Yet this is not to say that infertility is always more painful than cancer. The point is not to compare pain. Why enter the Suffering Olympics and compare our trials, competing for the gold medal for "most endured" and asserting that everybody else's stuff is meaningless unless we perceive that it's "as bad as mine"? The result is that no one acknowledges anyone else's pain.

Do you know someone who's in pain but haven't reached out to him or her because you're sure you're hurting more? Instead of contending for a medal in the Suffering Olympics, enter the *Special* Olympics—the race in which every participant helps everybody else make it to the finish line. And everybody wins.

Mike Justice exemplifies just such a model of comforting others. The associate pastor in a Texas church, Mike is visually impaired, to the point that he can barely tell the color of his wife's hair. Because of the effects of Mike's diabetes, he and his wife will never have children. And Mike is precisely the kind of person who would have every right to minimize others' pain. Yet he is the first to phone someone who has the flu and offer prayer support or provide empathy for tired young parents. Rather than letting a comparison of pain keep him from acknowledging another's hurt, he comforts people who are hurting and has a powerful ministry of encouragement as a result.

Know What You Need So You Can Ask for Help

While we wrestle with our longings, we have to figure out what to do with all the unsolicited advice that adds to the sting. In doing so, it's sometimes helpful to divide the world into two kinds of people: those who are trainable and those who aren't. Trying to train the untrainable might be as pointless as a circle. Those who are downright crass are probably beyond help. Many people, however, have good intentions but just say the wrong things. Understanding your own needs and desires will help you articulate what you need from them. Here are some ideas that may help you get started.

You need a silent, listening ear. Quiet presence is often the greatest comfort. During my first year of medical practice, I (Dr. Bill) sat with a couple who had lost a baby at twenty-three weeks' gestation. At a total loss for words, I sat in silence and wept with them. I felt surprised when they later thanked me profusely saying, "You said just the right words."
What words? I wondered.

You need others to acknowledge that your hurt is understandable. Sometimes it is hard to be around fertile friends. Their children are "grief triggers." It helps if they sometimes ask questions such as, "Does the very sight of my children cause you pain?" or "Do I talk about my kids too much?" It also helps if they see that their house full of kids means your friendship may go through a dry season. When making the guest list for baby showers, it helps if they ask, "Would you like to be invited, or would you prefer not to be?" You appreciate it if they write a note on the invitation that says, "I would love to have you there, but I would certainly understand if you choose not to come."

If they do talk about your infertility, you need them to keep it simple. Note that only one of the following statements is longer than six words: "I hope you're parents someday." "I'm sorry." "I'm here if you want to talk." "I feel sad for you." "How are you doing?" "May I hug you?" "It's okay to cry." "I love you."

You need the warmth of touch. A compassionate handshake, a pat on the back, a shoulder hug, or a bear hug go a long way. Martin Luther wrote, "We are all little Christs—when we touch, He touches."

You need them to accept your honest feelings. This goes beyond "allowing" you to cry. It also means letting you vent your anger from time to time. Anger in its various forms, from irritability to outbursts, is often part of the grief process.

The Bible is full of stories about people of faith who questioned God or got angry when life hurt. Moses wondered why God was so hard on him and requested, "If this is how you are going to treat me, put me to death right now—if I have found favor in your eyes—and do not let me face my own ruin" (Num. 11:15). Once Moses expressed himself, God came to his aid and met his need.

You need to hear that your mourning is justified. Statements such as "That must be hard" or "That's terrible" are far better than "It's not so bad" or "How can you feel that way?"

You need their prayers. Sometimes rather than saying, "I'll pray for you," (a promise that many fail to keep), it's better if your friends go pray and come back later to say, "I've been praying for you."

You need them to initiate acts of kindness. It's difficult for the person in pain to find the energy to figure out what he or she needs and then to ask for it. If others want to help, it's better if they make a specific offer rather than simply saying, "Call me if you need anything." They might ask, "What groceries can I pick up for you?" "Could I mow your lawn?" or, "May I bring dinner tonight?" One grieving man wrote, "I appreciated e-mail. I could read it when I felt like it and react freely. It's okay to yell at your computer."

You need them to be patient. Caring for people in pain takes energy, effort, and patience. Days may turn to months and even years, making it seem that the pain will never end. Patients and friends alike may grow weary of the long process you are going through. Sometimes it means hanging in there for what seems like forever.

What Can the Church Do on Mother's Day and Father's Day?

Following my miscarriage, for the first time I stayed home on Mother's Day. The following week a message in the church bulletin (placed there by my friends) said, "The altar flowers today are given with love and acknowledgement of all the babies of this church who were conceived on earth but born in heaven and for all who have experienced this loss."

Often the worst days of the year for an infertile person are Mother's Day and Father's Day ("M-Day" and "F-Day"). Going to a house of worship on such days can be like going to a house of mourning. Seeing all the corsages and boutonnieres is hard enough for an infertile person, but it's even more painful when all the mothers are asked to stand, as is the tradition in many churches. The only ones left sitting are children and those who wish they could have them. There are more productive ways to acknowledge the contributions parents make.

On these holidays, it's important that the church minister the grace of Christ by recognizing the pain in the pews. Consider writing to your pastor several weeks before these holidays. Ask that the church include in the bulletin or pastoral prayer mention of those for whom such days are painful. We encourage you to write a letter that looks something like this:

Dear [Pastor],

Father's Day is next Sunday. It's such a wonderful day for dads, and yet it's a difficult day for men experiencing infertility.

For one out of every six couples trying to have a baby, it's the impossible dream. That makes Father's Day an occasion for tears, not joy.

I'd like to ask that you please remember in your sermons and prayers those who have lost fathers, fathers who have lost children, fathers and children who are estranged from each other, and men who are unable to be fathers. It will not only comfort them; it will remind the fathers in our congregation who have been blessed that their children truly are wonderful gifts from God.

Warmly,

[Your name]

Understanding what comforts you will help you articulate what you need from others. In the process, you learn to ask others for help, and their caregiving skills improve. Thinking ahead about how to respond when confronted with yet another insensitive remark also helps you take a more proactive role in your own healing.

How to Handle Insensitive Comments

Be angry and sin not. Go ahead. Let yourself rant! Remember Job's sarcasm when he said, "Wisdom will die with you" (Job 12:2)? Feel free to privately gripe in the Spirit. When someone has made a stupid remark and you've managed once again to keep from being ugly, go ahead and throw a pillow when you get home.

Realize how easy it is to say insensitive things. An infertile woman noted, "I caught myself complaining about a sleepless night to a friend who had a sleep disorder and hadn't slept for more than five hours straight in more than a year. Another time I realized I'd bragged about my husband to a woman who had confided how much she longs to be married."

Give away grace. In Peter's second epistle, he admonishes his readers to "grow in grace" (2 Peter 3:18). Peter swore to Jesus that he would never deny him, but within hours, as Peter warmed himself by a fire, he made three such denials (Luke 22:54–60). After the resurrection, Jesus restored Peter. Standing by a fire where he'd cooked fish for breakfast, the Lord gave Peter three chances to declare his love (John 21:15–17). Peter understood what it was to receive grace.

Near the end of his life, Peter told his readers to grow in giving grace away. In the same way we've received God's grace, we're to dispense grace. That means giving others what they don't deserve, overcoming evil with good (Rom. 12:21).

Thank those who are truly comforting. At an infertility conference in Mexico, a young couple told of how they'd driven their neighbor to the hospital when she lost her baby at seven months' gestation. The couple had come to the conference on the eve of Mother's Day solely because they wanted to learn how to support their friend.

Sometimes it's easy to focus so much on the words that cause heartache that we fail to appreciate those in our lives who love us well, as this couple loved their neighbor. Take time to send a note of appreciation to those who show compassion or make an effort to understand your pain.

In his book *The Return of the Prodigal Son*, Henri Nouwen tells of a day he spent studying Rembrandt's painting by the same title. The painting is based on Jesus' parable, recorded in Luke 15, about the rebellious son whose father welcomes him home with dancing and a feast. Nouwen points out that we are eventually supposed to mature, going from being like the prodigal son, who receives grace, to being like the prodigal father, who is recklessly extravagant in giving grace away.

This means that while sometimes we educate others about our needs, other times we must simply throw up our hands and pray, "Father, forgive them; they don't know what they're saying." It means seeing a frazzled woman in a fit of impatience with her small children at the grocery store and saying to her, "You're having a hard day, aren't you?" Or when someone tells you about dreams shattered by multiple unplanned pregnancies, it means saying, "Fertility at either extreme is hard, isn't it?"

Most infertility patients can recite horror stories about the insensitive comments they've endured—the sister who announces in a singsong voice, "I got pregnant first!" The mother who badgers, "When are you going to give me grandchildren?" The brother-in-law who advises, "Hey, just take a vacation," or asks, "Want to borrow our kids?"

Being infertile is hard stuff. But it's also hard for the loved ones who fasten their seat belts for the roller-coaster ride while yet experiencing their own unique brand of pain. It's hard to watch loved ones hurt. Those who climb aboard and share the ride with us deserve gratitude, respect, and a little empathy now and then.

One infertility patient wrote about how life, with its many facets, can be especially hard. She was right.

- It's especially hard if you've never known what it's like to say, "I'm pregnant."
- It's especially hard if you've known the joy of being pregnant only to have it end in miscarriage.
- It's especially hard if you're single and you want to be married.
- It's especially hard if you're married and you want to present your spouse with a child but can't.
- It's especially hard if you have unplanned pregnancies and you have to bury your dreams.
- It's especially hard if you have no pregnancies and you have to bury your dreams.
- It's especially hard if you're an infertile woman, because infertility cuts to the core of your womanhood.
- It's especially hard if you're an infertile man, because infertility can feel like an attack on your virility.
- It's especially hard if you end up with six children after an IVF cycle.
- It's especially hard if your IVF cycle fails and all the embryos die.
- It's especially hard when tests show something's wrong but the treatments fail to correct it.
- It's especially hard if you have "unexplained infertility."
- It's just especially hard.

DISCUSSION QUESTIONS

1. What insensitive comments have you heard from others?
2. What insensitive comments have you made to people whose suffering has had a different shape from yours?
3. Make a list of the people in your life and what you need from them.
4. Who do you know who's "trainable," who might be a good source of support? What kind of training might help them? Consider lending them your copy of this book or ordering them a copy of the booklet *Understanding Infertility: Insights for Family and Friends* (available from Perspectives Press, www.perspectivespress.com).
5. What part of the infertility struggle do you find especially hard—medically, spiritually, relationally, and emotionally?
6. What complaints have you taken to God? Any? None? Take a few moments to do so now.
7. If someone has been especially sensitive to your pain, write and send him or her a thank-you note.

Chapter 6

WHERE IS GOD WHEN IT HURTS?

THE BIBLICAL INFERTILITY STORIES

I once again reconfirmed my faith, but found very little comfort in it. I knew only that I could not abandon it.

We have wondered at God's sovereignty. We have felt guilt that perhaps we were facing God's judgment for past sins.

Spiritual questions can cause the infertile couple more agony than the skyrocketing medical expenses, life on "hold," frustrating encounters at the physician's office, insurance hassles, and relational turmoil combined. In our dealings with thousands of infertility patients, only one said she never wondered if God might be punishing her. She was an atheist.

Suggestions from friends and spiritual leaders imply that infertility patients must be failing in some way. Those facing infertility wonder, "Where is God in our pain?" and, "Why does God let a teen conceive in the back of a Chevy while we—a couple longing for children—have to use a sperm wash in a sterile environment with a high-priced doctor and come up empty?"

Must We Multiply?

As early as Genesis 1, we read that God told Adam and Eve to "be fruitful and multiply." We read it and think this is something we can and *must* do. It seems we are unable to do the very thing for which we were created.

Weren't we created for procreation? That's how many people see God's command to the first couple to multiply—as a decree for all time.

Consider this message full of *erroneous* ideas, which we found on a website:

> There may be many factors involved in the reason "why" you're having problems conceiving, but none of them line up with God's will. How do I know? Because of Matthew 8:17 [he ... carried our diseases] and Genesis 1:28—where God tells mankind to be fruitful, multiply and fill the earth. We know God wouldn't have said this if he didn't know without a shadow of doubt that we could pull it off. God created humans to reproduce. Women were created to be able to have children. Men were created to be able to father children. If something has happened to change this, you can be sure that it isn't from God. Satan may be trying to prevent you from fulfilling Genesis 1:28, but he doesn't stand a chance if you're willing to stand on Matthew 8:17 and defeat this thing through faith. It isn't impossible, no matter what the doctors say. That is what I have received from the Lord, and I hope it helps someone to build their faith!

It seems that a failure to reproduce must mean God is coiling back to throw thunder and lightning to punish our lack of faith. We fear that he doesn't know or doesn't care about our problem. It seems we are unable to do the very thing for which we were created.

Although God gave Adam and Eve the command to be fruitful and multiply and later repeated the imperative for Noah (Gen. 9:7), in the New Testament we see an altogether different focus. In the New Testament, we see a change from the Old Testament's emphasis on physical multiplication to a focus on spiritual multiplication. Consider what the apostle Paul wrote to the Corinthian church about staying single: "I wish that all men were as I am [i.e., single]. But each man has his own gift from God; one has this gift, another has that. Now to the unmarried and the widows I say: It is good for them to stay unmarried, as I am" (1 Cor. 7:7–8). His reason for recommending single life over married life? So that men and women could live in undistracted service to the Lord. In other words, spiritual multiplication is even more important than physical multiplication. We are designed for more than human reproduction! According to current Jewish thought, if a couple is physically unable to have children, they are exempt from the command to reproduce.[1]

Should We Claim Promises?

Apparently, where childbearing is concerned, misapplication of Scripture abounds:

My favorite Scripture is Deuteronomy 7:14, "Thou shalt be blessed above all people: there shall not be male or female barren among you." This passage is referring, of course, to Israel, but I believe we can apply it to infertility as well.

I have been praying for children for almost fourteen years. One of those years, I decided to read the Bible through in a year. I took my high-lighter and marked every Scripture that could relate to being a promise for my children. Many of these Scriptures are Old Testament and were promised to Abraham's descendants. I claim these promises as mine, as well, based on Galatians 3:29, "And if ye be Christ's, then are ye Abraham's seed, and heirs according to the promise."

Anytime we read a promise in the Old Testament, we must consider the intended audience and determine whether those same promises actually apply to us. Often they don't. For example, God promised Sarah that he would bless her with a child. If Christians take the promise given to Sarah and claim that the same promise has been given to us, we're distorting what the text says. A promise made in the Bible to an individual is not a promise made to everybody for always. If your parents promised you a bike for Christmas, that promise applies to you and only you, not to your neighbor five generations from now.

The Lord promised military victory to Gideon if he would take an army of only three hundred men to war against a huge army (Judges 7:7). Modern military strategists wouldn't get far with such a small force. In the poetry of 1 Samuel 2:5, we read, "She who was barren has borne seven children." Should we claim this as a promise that God will give every infertile woman seven kids? No! It makes far more sense to understand that the timeless theological truth behind the promise is that God is able to bring about dramatic reversals of our circumstances.

Today, as Abraham's spiritual children, we inherit the *spiritual* promises given to him. We shouldn't read the promise to Abraham that he will father a great nation and assume we will each have a nation of physical children.

Is Infertility a Punishment?

Maybe this is a punishment for the things my husband and I did before we were married. We didn't have sex, but we "went too far." Or maybe it's a punishment because I took birth control pills. Or maybe it's because of the struggle I have with sins like eating too much.

In the Bible, Sarah and Hannah and Elizabeth prayed and got babies. So people told me, "I'm sure he'll be faithful to you—if you will just pray," and I used to believe them. Does that mean every infertile person lacks faith?

As we read through the Old Testament, we find places where it seems like the Bible says infertility is a curse. Some point to King David's wife, Michal, as an example (2 Sam. 6:23). Michal mocked David for dancing before the Lord and, as a result, was barren until her death. Yet if we look closely at her story, we see that we're not told that she *couldn't* conceive. We know only that she *didn't* conceive. Certainly God could have cursed her; the reason would have been clear. Yet another real possibility is that David simply stopped summoning her to the boudoir.

Still, when reading through the historical books one finds statements such as this:

> Then it shall come about, *because you listen to these judgments and keep and do them,* that the LORD your God will keep with you His covenant and His lovingkindness which He swore to your forefathers. He will love you and bless you and multiply you; He will also bless the fruit of your womb and the fruit of your ground, your grain and your new wine and your oil, the increase of your herd and the young of your flock, in the land which He swore to your forefathers to give you. You shall be blessed above all peoples; *there will be no male or female barren among you or among your cattle.*
>
> —Deuteronomy 7:12–14 NASB, italics ours

It's important to notice here that God was talking about infertility on a *national* scale rather than about individual cases. While this passage may seem to suggest that the faithful *will* all have children, that's not what it says. It speaks only of an epidemic that included even the animals. Later in the books of 1 and 2 Samuel, we see a national focus still in effect.

Beyond this, some people point to the *few* biblical examples of individual infertility associated with God's judgment and wrongly assume that *all* cases are a result of God's judgment. Note, however, that in these biblical examples, reasons for barrenness were limited to the following:

- An aunt and a nephew who slept together (Lev. 20:20).
- A man who married his brother's wife while the brother was still alive (Lev. 20:21).
- A female who committed adultery (Num. 5:20).

Moses listed these pronouncements under the Law, which the New Testament describes as the old covenant. Anyone who has trusted

Christ for salvation lives under a different—a new—covenant (Heb. 9:15). Today the primary focus of God's covenants has shifted from the nation to individuals in whom the Spirit dwells. And the focus has shifted from visible to spiritual realities. While the Old Testament events provide helpful instructions (1 Cor. 10:11), when we wrongly assume that the same system is in operation today, we grossly distort the truth.

We add to our misunderstanding of Scripture when we look up all the Bible references about infertility and then concoct a personal application. For example, we may see that everyone who prayed eventually got pregnant. This may lead us to assume that if we have faith, we too will get pregnant. We might notice all the barren women and assume that God views infertility as "a woman's problem."

So what are we *supposed* to learn from Sarah, Abraham's barren wife who finally conceived around age ninety? From Rachel, whose sister Leah was bearing all of their husband's kids? We can see that fertility became Rachel's god, so what can we glean from her story? Or from Samson's mother, who was infertile until an angel announced she was going to have a child? From Hannah, who prayed for a child?

First, it's important to note that *the infertility narratives in the Bible do not tell us all there is to know about infertility.* We need to see that the Bible stories describe exceptional circumstances. God was building a nation—physically and spiritually—against all odds. And infertility often serves to build tension within that narrative, making the story more compelling and prompting the reader to wonder how the Lord will pull off the impossible.

The Bible's infertility narratives were not written to teach principles about facing infertility per se. Yet they can provide much insight into the struggle of infertility and how God views it.

Abraham and Sarah: Is Anything Too Hard for the Lord?

We begin with the first infertile couple mentioned in the Bible: Sarah and Abraham. Calculate sometime how many cycles Sarah must have spent thinking, "Maybe this is the month," only to conclude, "Nope, this is *not* the month. Maybe next time." By her ninetieth birthday, she'd endured a lot of disappointment. In fact, she had quit "cycling." The text says, "Sarah was past the age of childbearing" (Gen. 18:11). What an understatement! Writer Calvin Miller notes that Sarah was probably the only woman ever to shop for Pampers and Depends in the same trip.

Yet God told Abraham, "Look up at the heavens and count the stars—if indeed you can count them. . . . So shall your offspring be" (Gen. 15:5). God promised Abraham numerous heirs, so he and his wife sought to bring about God's purposes in their own way. After waiting a long time, Sarah told Abraham to father a child (Ishmael) through a surrogate (Hagar), and as one Jewish writer has pointed out, "If you know the story, you know this lapse of faith produced the root of the Arab-Israeli conflict in the Middle East." Abraham and Sarah only did what many in their culture did, but they were supposed to be different.

Some have likened the Sarah-Abraham-Hagar arrangement to surrogacy. Yet a key difference is that the surrogate mother in modern arrangements doesn't marry the husband and live with the couple! Sadly, once Hagar was pregnant, she despised Sarah. And Sarah then blamed her husband for Hagar's ill treatment of her. What a mess!

Infertility pulls at such powerful forces in our souls that it's easy to have a "stop at nothing" mentality when seeking to fulfill those deep longings for a child. Thus, we must pause frequently and ask ourselves if we, too, are resorting to unethical—or, at the least, poorly thought-out—actions to bring about a happy ending. We may read Abraham's and Sarah's happy ending and focus so much on wanting to find a promise for ourselves that we miss the key question that the angel asked Sarah: "Is anything too hard for the LORD?" (Gen. 18:14).

Faith is not so much believing God *will* provide a child; rather, it's believing that nothing is too hard for him. And that involves believing that his ways, while mysterious, are trustworthy. He is still good, even if we don't have a biological child. If he knew it were the very best thing for us, he would cause us to conceive.

Isaac and Rebekah: God Answers Prayer

Next there's Isaac and Rebekah. The text tells us, "Isaac was forty years old when he married Rebekah. . . . Isaac prayed to the LORD on behalf of his wife, because she was barren. The LORD answered his prayer, and his wife Rebekah became pregnant" (Gen. 25:20–21). We learn later that Isaac was sixty when his twins were finally born (Gen. 25:26).

Are we to understand from these passages that infertility is the result of the husband's failure to pray? Such simplistic advice can bring immeasurable pain. Yet prayer is important. We read in the Bible about King Asa who, in the thirty-ninth year of his reign had a foot disease. The text says, "Though his disease was severe, even in his illness he did not seek help from the LORD, but only from the physicians" (2 Chron. 16:12). These biblical stories show us the priority of prayer, and also that physicians have limitations.

Sometimes God says no to our prayers because, in his omniscience, he has something better in mind for us in the long run. But sometimes we don't receive what we desire because we haven't asked. When our lives revolve around the doctor and his or her office hours, it's easy to trust in medicine rather than in the Lord. Rebekah and Isaac remind us to keep our focus on the Lord and his purposes.

In the writings of Ben Sira (38:1–9), often quoted in rabbinic literature and perhaps a source for James, we read the following words of wisdom that encourage balance: "Honor a physician with the honor due him for the uses which you may have of him: for the LORD created him. For of the most High comes healing. . . . The skill of the physician shall lift up his head: and in the sight of great men he shall be in admiration. The LORD has created medicines out of the earth; and he that is wise will not abhor them. . . . My son, in your sickness be not negligent: but pray unto the LORD, and he will make you whole."

Jacob and Rachel: What Do You Love Most?

Often when readers approach the story of Rachel and Leah (Genesis 29–30), they think of it primarily as an infertility story. But the point of the story is really to show how God built his nation, Israel. While God was accomplishing his purposes, the characters involved caused a lot of preventable heartache along the way. Yet he used even their sin to bring about his plan.

As the story goes, Jacob loved Rachel. But through his father-in-law's trickery, he married her less desirable sister, Leah, first. Seemingly to even the score, God granted Leah fertility, but Rachel was infertile. One got the love of a man; the other got the love of children. Before long, Leah had four boys and Rachel had none.

Rachel's pain is understandable, but she handled it badly. Rather than having mercy on her unloved sister, she envied her. Rachel blamed her pain on her husband, insisting, "Give me children, or else I die!" Jacob, outraged at the suggestion, asked, "Am I in the place of God, who has withheld from you the fruit of the womb?" (30:1–2 NKJV).

So Rachel decided to get children a different way. She gave Jacob her maid, Bilhah, who bore two sons. So Leah gave *her* servant to Jacob, who then had a total of four wives. Leah's maid birthed two kids, making the score Rachel–2, Leah–6.

One day Reuben, Leah's firstborn, then about ten years old, found some mandrakes and brought them to his mother. Today people tell infertile couples, "Just relax"; back then they said, "Go get some mandrakes." These plants were considered a fertility drug.[2]

Rachel told Leah, "I'll let you sleep with Jacob tonight in exchange for the mandrakes." She sold a night with her husband in exchange for the "magic fertility potion."

When Jacob came home, Leah went skipping out to him and told him that she'd bought a night with him. So Jacob had sex with her, and she conceived a fifth son. Then Leah said, "God has given me my hire because I gave my maid to my husband" (30:18, my translation). Leah didn't say God had blessed her because she hired her husband with mandrakes, which is what we might expect. Rather, she believed that God was blessing her for giving her maid to Jacob.

Rachel had acted out of superstition by putting so much stock in the mandrakes' ability to cure her infertility. And ironically, the mandrakes provided Leah with an opportunity to conceive again. Leah went on to have two more children, so the score was Rachel–2, Leah–9. God made it clear to Rachel that children don't come from using mandrakes. As we read on, we see that our "idols" can be the very things that destroy us.

Eventually God allowed Rachel to have the long-awaited child. We might expect her to name him something like, "God is good," but instead she named him Joseph, whose name is a play on the word "add." Rachel said, "May the LORD *add* to me another son!" (30:24, italics ours). When God gave her what she wanted, she missed the gratitude stage and went straight to craving more.

Rachel did go on to have another child, Benjamin. But she died giving birth to him. The very thing that consumed her in life took her life; that which became more important to her than God destroyed her.

How often is that true of us?

The decade-plus catfight between Rachel and Leah increased their misery. Yet God still accomplished his grander purposes: through these women, the twelve tribes of Israel came into being. Regardless of the sinful attitudes and actions involved, Rachel and Leah were instruments of God. Later in the Bible, when Boaz announced he would marry Ruth, the villagers pronounced a blessing on her, saying, "May the LORD make [her] ... like Rachel and Leah, who together built the house of Israel" (Ruth 4:11). Rachel and Leah are remembered not for their bickering but for how God accomplished his ultimate will through them.

We Westerners like a good love story, so we tend to root for Rachel because she and Jacob were in love. And infertile people identify more with her pain than that of Leah's. Yet the author paints Leah as being more of a hero than Rachel. Some of the names Leah chose for her children demonstrated her faith. We may even think of Rachel's son Joseph, the one with the coat of many colors, as the son of promise, but it was Judah through whom David and ultimately Jesus Christ would come. And Judah was a son of the "other wife," Leah.

No matter how we handle our infertility, we can never thwart God's purposes. Yet unlike Leah and Rachel, we can prevent ourselves and others from suffering additional misery along the way.

The Nameless Infertile Woman: "Pay Attention to *All* That I Said"

Fast-forward to the time right before the era when kings reigned in Israel. God himself was the leader of the people, and he led them through deliverers, or judges. In Judges 13, we find the story of one such deliverer—Samson. Before he was born, his mother, described only as "the wife of Manoah," was infertile.

During this time in history, the nation engaged in all sorts of evil acts. Thus, the Lord let Israel's enemies conquer them for forty years. But finally he decided it was time to intervene. So his angel appeared to Manoah's wife with some news. He told her that she'd have a son who was not supposed to drink alcohol or shave his head. But then he added something very important: "And he shall begin to deliver Israel from the hands of the Philistines" (13:5 NASB).

When Manoah's wife told her husband what had happened, she left out the "deliverer" part. So Manoah asked God to send the angel back to provide more information. The angel reappeared, and when Manoah asked him about his son's vocation and mode of life, the angel said only, "Let the woman pay attention to all that I said" (13:13 NASB). Manoah's wife was so focused on having a baby that she missed the bigger spiritual picture.

In biblical times, when a writer avoided naming someone, as he did here with "Manoah's wife," it was usually to avoid honoring that person. It signals the reader that the unnamed character has failed in some way. For Manoah's wife, the good news about having a baby overshadowed God's more important plans. And for many couples caught in the swirl of infertility, it's easy for all thoughts, energies, and resources to go into the quest to reproduce. Or maybe the number one focus is doing anything to make one's partner happy so life can feel normal again. These may be important goals, but they are not the *most* important. Manoah's wife missed the grand spiritual impact of what God was accomplishing in the history of his people because she was so focused on having a baby. It's still possible today to be so focused on completing the personal family portrait that we miss God's larger purposes.

Hannah—Worship the Fertility God or the God of Fertility?

The most in-depth biblical picture we get of infertility comes through Hannah (1 Sam. 1–2:11). Like Samson's mother, Hannah lived during the time of the judges. At that time, the people of Israel were so decadent that a concubine traveling with her master was raped and abused all night by a group of men and then left dead on the doorstep. Her master took her home, cut her into twelve pieces, and sent the parts to all the areas of Israel (Judges 19:29–30). If ever Israel needed a godly leader, it was then.

Enter Hannah. She was married to Elkanah, a man with two wives. Back then, husbands often took second wives to produce heirs in the event of infertility, as is still practiced in some cultures today. Why? They had no social security, public safety officials, or relief organizations to care for the needs of the poor. They also had no hospitals or nursing homes. A couple's entire future and well-being depended on offspring to feed them, support them, and protect them in their old age. Imagine the suffering infertility brought!

Hannah and her husband worshiped God, while the people around them offered sacrifices to the local Baal. Picture an infertile woman refusing to worship Baal. Can't you just hear her neighbors? "You've enraged the fertility god!"

To make matters worse, Penninah, the superfertile "other wife," provoked Hannah to the point that she wept and refused to eat. Then her husband, suffering from a clear case of "testosteronesia," asked, "Hannah, why do you weep? Why do you not eat? And why is your heart grieved? Am I not better to you than ten sons?" (1:8 NKJV).

As is so often the case, words intended to comfort his wife only polarized the couple. More than anything, he wanted his wife's happiness; more than anything, she wanted a baby. No doubt Hannah felt isolated. How could her husband comprehend her pain? He, on the other hand, did all he could to show her his love. What else could he do?

Many husbands have said words similar to Elkanah's. They ask, "Am I not enough? Even if we never have children, I love you. Don't you love me? What about me?"

Hannah prays in bitterness of soul with anguished tears. Then she makes a vow that if God will give her a male child, she will give him back to the Lord. Even the priest doesn't "get it." When he sees her lips moving in prayer, he thinks she's drunk.

Notice in this story that Hannah has a normal stress response to infertility: she cries, feels depressed, won't eat, sees things differently from her husband, and prays in anguish. Yet God does not say, "Stop obsessing!" Instead, the text says, "The LORD remembered her" (1:19). That word "remembered" means he answered her prayer.

Yet the story doesn't end there. We find, once again, that God intends something greater than curing infertility. Often we observe that

Hannah got what she wanted but fail to see what it cost her to keep her vow. When her son was a toddler, she said, "Now I give him to the LORD" (1:28). Then she penned a lovely hymn proclaiming, "There is no one holy like the LORD!" (2:2). She saw her son only once a year—an astounding sacrifice on her part. So it cost Hannah a lot to be part of what God was doing.

We see in Hannah a woman who trusted God through the pain. And his ultimate answer required sacrifice on Hannah's part. Yet she depended on him and obeyed. Against the dark backdrop of sin in the nation, when it looked like God had walked out on the nation in disgust, her son, Samuel, the prophet, came as a bright light.

Elizabeth: No Shame

An infertile woman was touring the cathedrals of Europe, and she noticed that everywhere she went, icons of Mary were brightly lit with numerous pilgrims' candles. She also noted that images of Elizabeth always seemed neglected, dimly lit by whatever natural light made it through the stained-glass windows. This tourist, feeling a special affinity with infertile Elizabeth, bought all the candles in one of the cathedrals. Then, as the woman described it, "I departed with a smile, having left 'my friend Liz' in a blaze of glory."

We read Elizabeth's story in Luke 1:5–25. She and her husband were old and childless when an angel appeared to her husband, a priest, and announced that Elizabeth would have a baby. When Elizabeth conceived, she remained in seclusion for five months. "The Lord has done this for me," she said. "In these days he has shown his favor and taken away my disgrace *among the people*" (1:25, italics ours).

In biblical times, fertile women often looked down on infertile women. Sarah was despised by her Egyptian servant, Hagar, when Hagar conceived and her mistress couldn't (Gen. 16:4). The same thing happened to Hannah when Elkanah's second wife conceived (1 Sam. 1:6–7). Notice that Elizabeth's disgrace is "among the people" and not "in the sight of God."

Note, too, how often the miracle child in these narratives ends up being used by God to lead his people. Rather than being a punishment for sin, in the biblical texts, infertility is often an affliction of the *righteous*.

For some infertility patients, understanding that God is under no obligation to provide a child can bring relief as they see that they are not being punished after all. That was the case for a patient who wrote this:

The turning point was when I came to understand that my infertility was not a punishment from God. I figured that I did some bad things during my late teens that I was being punished for. But I was finally able to see that God did have a plan for whatever reason, and right then it didn't include a child.

For other patients, this understanding can come as a huge jolt when they suddenly realize they are not guaranteed a child. At a recent symposium, Dr. Bill gave a lecture on "Infertility and Spirituality." Afterward a woman pulled him aside and, with tears in her eyes, asked, "You mean even if I obey all his commands, I might not get a baby?" With grace and compassion, he helped her to see that such a clear cause-and-effect relationship was not promised to her.

A seminary professor and his wife who are unable to have children pour their lives into their students. A pastor and his wife came from Africa to the United States, went through an in vitro fertilization (IVF) cycle, and ended up with twins. Another Christian couple tried IVF, and when that didn't work, they adopted.

In each of these cases, the couple was more committed to knowing and loving God—to pursuing him—than they were to having a child. Does that mean they didn't agonize? No. Does that mean they didn't complain bitterly to him? Of course not. Does that mean they never argued with him? No way.

But in the end, they knew it all boiled down to two questions: Is God good? Will I trust him? How we answer those two questions may be the most important part of the infertility journey.

"Haven't I Earned a Child?"

Much of life is cause and effect, so it's easy to let the mentality that we've earned a child creep into our view of God and the Christian life. We think that if we do certain things—right things—*voilà!* God will bless us with wealth, children, and whatever else we might want. So we establish a mentality of entitlement. We think, "If I go to church, read my Bible, pray—*bingo!* God is honor-bound to bless me with a child." When the nursery stays empty, we wonder why we failed to get our prize when we have put our dollar of obedience into the machine. We think that either the machine is broken or we are.

It's so unjust! My best friend got pregnant before she was married. She and her now-husband just announced she is pregnant again. They leave their daughter at daycare and live in low-income apartments. But my husband and I "waited until we were married," and I can stay home. Yet God chooses to bless them, not us.

We both became believers early in life, we were leaders in our church youth group, I was enrolled in seminary preparing for a life of ministry, I was licensed and ordained, I've taught Sunday school classes, and I have even been the pastor of a church. Theologically, we have all our ducks in a row.... If we were compiling a resume of why God ought to give us children, we felt that we had adequate qualifications.

Job's friends had just such a cause-and-effect view of life, and it got them into trouble. They assumed Job was suffering because he must have done something awful. Later God told them that they had not spoken rightly about him, as Job had. Ultimately justice prevails, but not always in this life.

Those who have eternal life in knowing Jesus Christ (John 3:16) have the promise that God will never leave us (Heb. 13:5). And God's presence is the greatest thing in all of life, because it is the *only* thing that brings true, lasting soul satisfaction. We have no promise that he will give us any temporal benefits. And even if God does answer the prayer for children, those blessings will never satisfy us at the deepest levels of our souls.

Only intimacy with the Father through the Son satisfies the soul's deepest longings.

DISCUSSION QUESTIONS

1. Discuss with your spouse the spiritual impact that infertility has on each of you.
2. What kind of spiritual assistance is available to you in your faith community? In the community in general?
3. Do you feel your personal spiritual walk has progressed, stalled, or disappeared during treatment? Explain.
4. Have you ever considered walking away from your faith? Have there been times when you felt like giving up on God? Describe why.
5. What quotes in this chapter best express where you are on your spiritual journey?

Chapter 7

THE SPIRITUAL STRUGGLE

IS INFERTILITY A CURSE?

People at church say, "Maybe it's not God's will for you to be parents." You pray and feel as if your requests never go any higher than the ceiling. You wonder why God says no to fulfilling your deepest longings. You ask what you are supposed to do with your life. You ponder whether God really has the power to heal your body and if he has the mercy to care. Or perhaps you find faith where before you had none. You discover internal resources you never knew you had. Or maybe you doubt and have faith at the same time. Spiritual responses to infertility are as varied as the patients themselves.

Tragic as it was for us to lose the pregnancy, I never questioned my faith or felt abandoned. If anything, I've grown in Christ because of my loss. I've found comfort and solace in my faith. The loss is devastating, but through prayer I can speak to God about my anger and depression. I did have trouble returning to church, though. I found it hard to sit through infant dedications and baptisms. But I never tried to hide my feelings. I've cried openly. No matter what happens to me, God is always there.

I haven't really questioned my faith, but I have certainly asked God why he didn't make things right for me.

For infertility patients, the grief of lost dreams brings added despair over losing faith in God's goodness. And sometimes the latter comes from misunderstanding or misapplying the very book intended to draw us into closer fellowship with God. Consider Jennifer's story:

An acquaintance gave me a gift—a devotional for pregnant women. She had no idea I was going through fertility testing. Later I had a laparoscopy during which doctors removed a fallopian tube. But I believed, reflecting on the book, that the Lord had "told" me that I was going to be pregnant. Later a man who said he was gifted in "prophetic prayer" prayed that I was going to be a mother of a number of children. Was this another promise from the Lord?

What if he really hadn't promised me? I sought counsel to see if I was crazy for having such faith in this "promise." My counselors made me consider that I may not have received a promise at all. I can't help but wonder if the Lord allowed this "mistake" so that I could trust in him until I was more able to handle the truth.

In the last chapter, we surveyed some of the stories of infertile people in the Bible. In this chapter, we'll consider some Bible verses that get pulled out of context and mishandled. As Jennifer's story demonstrates, having a right understanding of what God says about himself and about our struggle helps us have both realistic expectations and a clear understanding of how deeply he cares.

Sing, O Barren—Nation?

Around 700 B.C., the prophet Isaiah wrote words of warning to the nation of Israel because of their sin. But he prophesied that following the times of judgment, they'd experience blessing. To describe the blessing, he uses the metaphor of the nation as a childless wife: "'Sing, O barren woman, you who never bore a child; burst into song, shout for joy, you who were never in labor; because more are the children of the desolate woman than of her who has a husband,' says the LORD" (Isa. 54:1).

Whether in internet chat rooms or at conferences, many infertile people have spoken of "claiming this promise." They have interpreted it as clear evidence that they will conceive, and they've encouraged other patients to claim it as well. This represents a fundamental misuse of literature, not to mention of Scripture. The Old Testament prophets often likened the nation of Israel to a bride, with God as her groomsman.

By plucking one verse out of its context, we can make the Bible say anything we want it to say. Our Western mindset tends to focus excessively on the individual, and we want a personal word from God. We want a direct sign or prediction that he will bless us with a child. We want to gaze into the future. Out of that desire, we may take texts that address a nation and apply them to our own circumstances. Doing so often comforts us, as we believe that according to his own word, God *must* bless us. Yet it also sets us up for disillusionment with God when he doesn't deliver the so-called promise.

What Is the Desire of Your Heart?

Having children is not a right; but having children is a nearly universal desire. When they hear the word "desire," many so-called comforters quote Psalm 37:4: "Delight yourself in the LORD and he will give you the desires of your heart."

Often childless couples hear this and assume that if they will delight in God, they are guaranteed a child. In response, a few conjure up some external "proof" that they have spiritual priorities. One woman volunteered for nursery duty at church. Another spoke of "cutting a deal" with God by promising to be the perfect, godly mother if he would deliver.

Psalm 37 as a whole describes the falsehood of believing that the virtuous are immediately rewarded and the evil are immediately punished. The psalmist cautions us against discontentment such as one patient described:

> *My husband is annoyed with a woman at church. She married an unbeliever and now has five children. Her husband doesn't work, and they live with her parents. She just announced she's pregnant again! Real fair God, real fair. More than anything my relationship with Christ has suffered during our infertility. It has shaken my faith from top to bottom!*

In the context of precisely this kind of injustice, the psalmist encourages the reader to trust in God's goodness despite the seemingly contradictory evidence. The message: usually if we wait long enough, we will see the righteous vindicated and the evil punished.

This psalm is poetry. So we must hesitate to read it as *promise*. This patient got it right:

> *After my miscarriage I pondered the meaning of "Delight yourself in the Lord and he will give you the desires of your heart" (Ps. 37:4). I had always read that as a promise. Then I began to see that many of the Psalms and Proverbs are generalized truths, not guarantees. And I knew that if I fully delighted myself in him, he—and not a child— would be the ultimate desire of my heart, anyway.*

A similar misunderstanding comes from taking out of context all the statements about God hearing and answering prayer. Some conclude that if they pray and then don't get a child, either God is unfaithful or it is their fault for somehow lacking faith. Yet often even when we have faith, God says wait, and even no.

Children Are *a* Gift

Behold, children are a gift of the LORD,
The fruit of the womb is a reward.

—Psalm 127:3 NASB

This verse has brought pain for many infertile couples. They wonder why they've failed to receive such a "reward" while so many unmarried teens and abusive parents have won the prize.

The word "children" is actually "sons"—the idea being not that boys are better than girls but that in the culture of the time, boys provided protection and economic potential.

"Gift/reward" would be better translated as "inheritance/wages." It's not like a prize for good behavior; it's more like an unmerited economic windfall. At the time the psalmist wrote this, the concept of having a pension was nonexistent. Picture a world much like the Old West. If you had a big ranch, you needed a posse of sons to ensure justice for your family. The more sons, the more physically and financially secure you were.

Today those of us with insurance, alarm systems, access to legal counsel, a police force, and a host of other means of security have most of the benefits the psalmist had in mind here. In fact, having no children often means having more of these things. In an agrarian culture, children bring financial security. In an industrialized culture, children are often the opposite; they're expensive! It's important to see, too, that children are *a* gift from the Lord, but they are not the only, or even the ultimate, means of blessing.

Saved through Childbearing?

But [a woman or wife] will be saved through childbearing—if they continue in faith, love and holiness with propriety.

—1 Timothy 2:15

An infertility patient was reading along in her Bible when she came upon this verse. She broke out in a cold sweat, fearful that she could never go to heaven if she didn't have children. That is certainly *not* what this text is saying. But the reader was in good company in having trouble with it. Some scholars say this is the hardest verse in the Bible to understand.

Let's clarify what it does *not* mean. The apostle Paul, writing to his protégé, Timothy, is talking about women (probably wives) learning and teaching, not about eternal life. Interpreting this passage as saying that women have to bear children to get to heaven would contradict Jesus' and Paul's own teachings elsewhere: salvation is by grace through faith, not by any works we have done. It would also contradict Paul's teaching in 1 Corinthians 7, where he elevates the state of singleness.

Paul speaks here of Adam and Eve and the Fall. He may mean that, despite Eve's influence on Adam to sin (she messed up), womankind is saved—that is, sanctified—through either the birth of Christ ("the" childbearing) or through the role of mothering. In this case, "women" would not refer to women as individuals but to women as a class.

We know that Paul's respect for women was unrelated to their ability to bear children. For example, he continually mentioned Priscilla and Aquila in his epistles, calling them his partners in ministry. He also highly esteemed Phoebe (Rom. 16:1–2). In neither case are these women's biological relationships ever mentioned.[1]

A patient told us, "The idea that even if I can't have children, I should be a *spiritual* mother has come as a totally new concept. It had never occurred to me that I need to be nurturing the next generation, whether or not I have my own kids."

It's Only Natural

> *There are three things that will not be satisfied,*
> *Four that will not say, "Enough":*
> *Sheol, and the barren womb,*
> *Earth that is never satisfied with water,*
> *And fire that never says, "Enough."*
> —Proverbs 30:15–16 NASB

> *I was able to move toward acceptance of God's plan for my life only after realizing the truth in Proverbs 30. It compares the barren womb to other powerful forces of nature, and for the first time I really felt that God knew—that he not only accepted me with all my "crazy" emotions, but he created me to have them and he understood the way they affected me.*

Proverbs 30:15–16 is probably one of the least-quoted Scriptures about infertility, but it is perhaps one of the most profound. "Sheol" is "the grave" or "death" in the Old Testament. It is personified here with other natural forces as entities that can speak. If they could talk, they would never say, "I'm satisfied; I need no more." That is, death would never say, "No one else can die because I'm content that the underworld is full." In the same way, after it has rained, the earth eventually soaks up the water that has accumulated on its surface. And a fire, unless it runs out of fuel, will not stop simply because it has burned enough.

The barren womb is considered to have a force parallel to these natural forces. It is perfectly natural for the childless couple to desire children and to feel unsatisfied when that desire goes unmet. Such longing—such lack of being content or satisfied—is the natural order of things.

God understands! He's the one who set up such natural laws. Desiring children is a good and natural desire, and when conception does not occur, it's devastating. God does not minimize such pain; in fact, he appears to validate it.

Sometimes God has grander purposes in allowing suffering than what we might think. Why would he make us a certain way and then withhold the very thing he made us to yearn for? A glance through the entire Bible demonstrates that there are numerous reasons why God allows pain. What follows is an overview of some of these reasons. But we warn you that while you're in the midst of the fire, these explanations will not quench the flames. They are things people have told us in retrospect about their infertility experience.

Why God Allows Suffering

To Punish Sin

Often our first thought is to think, as these patients have, that our pain must be happening because of God's judgment:

> I've had two miscarriages. With the first one, I was young and drinking a lot. The second time, I stopped everything when I found out I was pregnant. I still lost the baby. What have I done that was so bad that God would punish me so horribly? That was almost six months ago, but I still can't figure out why.

> The feeling of punishment came, mixed with anger. I'd already endured sexual abuse, so I felt angry for being "punished" all my life. The sense of injustice is greater because the abuser has a beautiful and sound daughter—like the daughter I always dreamed I'd have. So I wrote an "Indignant Letter to God." I said I was tired of being punished for something—I didn't know what. I told him I'd had enough.

These patients thought God was punishing them. And certainly God sometimes directs or allows events to bring justice where wrong has been done. Such was the case in the Old Testament (described in Lev. 20:20–21) for an Israelite who slept with his aunt or sister-in-law. We may not have done anything as awful as sleeping with an in-law, yet we recognize that we are sinners standing before a holy God. When we see life from that perspective, we ask with the psalmist, "If you, O LORD, kept a record of sins, O Lord, who could stand?" (Ps. 130:3).

We do owe God a debt we could never pay on our own—the penalty for sinning and offending a holy God. Yet his perfect Son, as our substitute, has paid the debt so we could go free. All we must do is receive God's free offer of eternal life through his Son. Several patients we've met have crossed the bridge from unbelief to faith as a direct result of their infertility.

Nevertheless, Jesus warned against always seeing a direct link between sin and suffering. He asked his disciples, "Those eighteen who died when the tower in Siloam fell on them—do you think they were more guilty than all the others living in Jerusalem?" (Luke 13:4). A modern equivalent might be, "Do you think all those killed on September 11 were worse sinners than the rest of us?" The implied answer is no!

The Bible makes it clear that the Father does not punish those whom he has adopted through their relationship with his Son. He may discipline them (Heb. 12:8), but he also promises that if they confess, they will be forgiven (1 John 1:9).

When Jesus' disciples saw a blind man, they asked Jesus, "Rabbi, who sinned, this man or his parents, that he was born blind?"

"Neither this man nor his parents sinned," Jesus said, "but this happened so that the work of God might be displayed in his life" (John 9:2–3). Then he healed the man.

This leads us to the next reason God allows suffering.

To Display God's Work

Maybe God is trying to bless us in some other way, or maybe he is trying to teach me something. Or maybe this is from Satan, and God is just choosing to let it happen. I don't know. At this point, I don't know where God stands on my infertility!

Consider what happened to the apostle Paul, one of the greatest heroes of the faith ever to live. He had an affliction that he called his "thorn in the flesh." We don't know if it was a person who persecuted him, bad eyesight, or poor health. But whatever it was, he longed for God to remove it.

"Three times I pleaded with the Lord to take it away from me," Paul wrote.

But the Lord said no. He told Paul, "My grace is sufficient for you, for my power is made perfect in weakness."

The apostle concluded, "Therefore I will boast all the more gladly about my weaknesses, so that Christ's power may rest on me. That is why, for Christ's sake, I delight in weaknesses, in insults, in hardships,

in persecutions, in difficulties. For when I am weak, then I am strong"
(2 Cor. 12:8–10).

> *It didn't occur to me in the early stages of my infertility that God was
> using it to build his kingdom, that maybe my womb was closed for a
> good reason. I'll never forget discovering that God, at times, closed an
> individual's womb for corrections, instruction, or edification. Wham!
> I finally got it. My womb was not closed as punishment at all. God
> wanted me to use my infertility to bring glory to him through it. That
> day I got on my knees and gave my infertility to God. "Lord," I prayed,
> "you know our desire to become parents. You know the pain and the
> struggle I go through every day with this disappointment, but I trust
> in you Father, that if your plan includes my womb to be closed at this
> time, then I can deal with it."*

Consider that those around you are watching how you respond to
this heartache. Maybe your suffering is not about your own failure to
learn what you're supposed to learn. Perhaps God has allowed your
pain to demonstrate his sufficient grace in and through your life to
someone who needs an encounter with his supernatural power. Maybe
you can comfort others through the information you learn (2 Cor. 1:3).

To Draw Us to God

Jacqueline, a cancer patient who died in 2001, did not have a relationship with the Lord until she got the diagnosis of cancer. A friend
gave her a book in which she read about God's holiness and love. Later
Jacqueline wrote, "I thank him daily for giving me cancer, as it was his
way to bring me to him. Even if cancer takes my life, it will never take
my soul."[2]

What about you? Do you look at a sunset, see his power, and long
to have fellowship with God? If so, first admit to him that you fall short
of his perfect standard of holiness (Rom. 3:23). Then acknowledge that
Jesus, in his love, died as the perfect substitute, taking your place to bear
the penalty you deserved (Rom. 5:8). Finally, simply tell him, "Thank
you for your amazing grace. Help me to know you better."

To Give Us Something Better

During the same dark period in Israel's history in which Hannah
lived, we find Ruth. She lived with her husband in Moab, Israel's next-
door neighbor. The national deity in Moab was Chemosh, and histori-
ans say worshipers of Chemosh offered human sacrifices.

Ruth and her husband were married ten years with no child being
born, which suggests a fertility problem. Then her husband and his

brother and father died, leaving Ruth with only her sister-in-law and her mother-in-law, Naomi—three widows with no protection. So Ruth accompanied Naomi back to her original home in Bethlehem.

Once there, Ruth worked daily in the fields of Naomi's relative, Boaz, a prominent man in town. Before long, Boaz instructed his servants to help Ruth. When word got back to Naomi about it, she sent Ruth to propose marriage to Boaz, a man who was much older than Ruth. Boaz was flattered by the young woman's willingness to marry him and was impressed with her selflessness of putting her mother-in-law's needs for security above her own desire for a love match. So Boaz married Ruth. And their grandchildren turned out to include King David and ultimately the Messiah, Jesus Christ (see Matt. 1:5–16).

We see from this story that Ruth was childless for ten years in a culture that offered children as human sacrifices. Then she lost her husband and all her security. Yet after all those losses, she went on to have both a child and a name that will last forever. Sometimes God withholds what we want most so that he can later give us something even better.

It's a Mystery

The book of Job provides us with some insight into one more reason why God allows suffering. The Lord gives Job a little quiz that illustrates the huge gulf between human intelligence and God's:

> "Have you ever given orders to the morning, or shown the dawn its place, that it might take the earth by the edges and shake the wicked out of it? . . .
>
> "Have you journeyed to the springs of the sea or walked in the recesses of the deep? Have the gates of death been shown to you? Have you seen the gates of the shadow of death? Have you comprehended the vast expanses of the earth? Tell me, if you know all this.
>
> "What is the way to the abode of light? And where does darkness reside?"
>
> —Job 38:12–13, 16–19

We flunked the quiz. How about you? Is it any wonder that our suffering makes no sense to us? Since God is that far beyond us, of course we can't understand. So ultimately the answer to the why question is this: It's a mystery.

A colleague who died of brain cancer once noted, "When God allows us to suffer, it's not a detour; it's part of the main road (Prov. 20:24). We may not know the reason for our suffering, but we know that suffering comes to accomplish God's purpose. As a sovereign and good God, he is not taken by surprise when his children suffer. Rather than being thwarted, his purposes advance through our suffering."

Knowing that God is sovereign doesn't mean we must have dry eyes and respond with passivity to prove we have faith. It means we rest in the assurance that he's in control, despite our pain. We know he is able to open and close the human womb. Infertility comes as no surprise to him, and he has to allow this suffering to happen for it to touch anyone.

Therein lies the tension, though. God is all-loving, yet he allows this pain; God is all-powerful, yet he doesn't take away the hurt. So we ask: "Is God good?" and "Will I trust him?" These are the most important questions we can ask and answer on the infertility journey.

DISCUSSION QUESTIONS

1. What does your suffering mean to you? Have you tried to find some significance in it? Have others tried to tell you why you're suffering?
2. Does God feel far away, near, or both? Explain.
3. Have you ever thought God promised you a child? What do you think now?
4. Sometimes when people read about biblical reasons for suffering, they initially find the explanations highly spiritual-sounding, unhelpful, even hurtful. Is that how you feel now? Did any of the quotes encourage you? Did any seem to fit your situation?
5. Have you ever prayed acknowledging Christ's payment for your sins? If not, what keeps you from doing so now?
6. Do you know of anyone whose life you can touch with the gospel as a result of your pain? Describe how.
7. How have you grown through your infertility experience? How has your spouse grown?
8. How might you support someone who is hurting spiritually?
9. Who in the next generation can you mentor as a spiritual parent—not in order to bargain with God, but for no other reason than for that person's benefit?
10. What are some of life's seeming injustices that you find most difficult to accept? Spend some time talking to God about them, expressing your thoughts and frustrations.
11. Is God good? Can you trust him?

Chapter 8

THE UNDERLYING QUESTION

WHY DID GOD CREATE SEX?

When we first started trying to conceive, sex was fabulous. Then I kept getting my period . . .

Sex is a dreaded event—as enjoyable as shoveling snow off the driveway.

I got pregnant after we adopted. Everybody said, "See, you adopted and then you got pregnant—you must have relaxed." But I got pregnant through intrauterine insemination (IUI). We don't do sex; infertility ruined that for us.

Some say "sex and the infertile couple" is an oxymoron. As if the absence of a child weren't enough, most infertile couples report a dramatic decrease in their level of sexual pleasure. How sad, even ironic, that the contact designed to result in oneness, and ultimately a child, becomes a chore.

We began to consider lovemaking senseless at any time other than "the time"—viewing our marriage strictly as a baby-making enterprise.

Finally the test said we should get together. But then another problem arose . . . actually it didn't arise—that was the problem. I like having sex, and I like having sex with my wife. I just find it difficult to perform on schedule. It got so bad that we had to go to a therapist.

Our sex life suffered. Sometimes I felt like a baby-making machine rather than a man. At times I would avoid sex when we were supposed to. My wife would either beg or demand me to perform, making things worse. Sex was a job.

If my husband called himself my "egg slave" or "robot," another woman's spouse dubbed himself her "trained seal." Alone, and with our husbands, we [try] to cope while muddling through mechanical, timed sex. . . . Deeply sweet but trying to retain his manhood, my own husband glumly referred to our lovemaking as "egg duty." As in, "Do I have egg duty tonight, or is it tomorrow?" At first I was resentful— considering all that I was putting up with, out of his sight—but then I decided to commiserate with him in his own sad language. "Oh, you poor thing," I'd say, "you must be an egg slave tonight."[1]

I just say, "I got the shot," and he knows that it's "time." My friend's husband is more touchy, so she uses nonverbal signals. When she's ready to ovulate, she hangs her nightgown on their bedroom doorknob.

Want to know what's sad? Now we do the wild thing and experience REM sleep at the same time.

My man "rose to the occasion" while doped up on morphine, hooked up to an IV pole, trying to pass a kidney stone. Loving? Absolutely! Sexy? No way.

Sex usually loses its magic during infertility treatment, because it must be executed or withheld regardless of mood. Men feel pressured to perform at optimal, doctor-directed times. As keepers of the ovulation kits and bearers of the clinic's news, women give the cues. Many couples invent code words and phrases ("trained seal," "egg duty") to communicate about the nonerotic process. Some husbands who want to avoid forced intimacy prefer simply to deliver their sperm to the clinic, where their waiting wives are artificially inseminated. One woman reports that, while she's endured surgery to conceive, her husband won't even make the effort to engage in physical contact at ovulation time.

The result: ruined sex lives litter the infertility landscape.

How can a couple, whose love life now has the privacy of a celebrity wedding, return to lovemaking that's about intimacy? One way is to create a dichotomy between two different kinds of sex: *lovemaking* sex and *baby-making* sex.

It's sort of like taking two kinds of trips—the slow route and the fast route. The two are as different as gondolas and powerboats. When you take a gondola, you enjoy the scenery; when you take the powerboat, you cruise full steam ahead to reach your destination as rapidly as possible.

Every June my (Sandi's) family gathers at the Oregon coast for group camping. Inevitably we load up a van full of relatives and drive down Route 101, the old coast highway. We may take five hours to cover fifty miles as we stop to catch crabs or hit ice-cream shops.

About fifty miles inland lies another highway. Interstate Highway 5 (I-5) cuts through Pacific West Coast terrain from northern Washington to Tijuana, Mexico. An eight-lane divided highway, I-5 is the way to go if you want to make good time. Each highway has its function. But you don't take Route 101 when you want to make the Mexican border by lunchtime.

Lovemaking sex is like the coast route; you savor the sensual experience. Baby-making sex is like I-5; you get the job done. Fast. Not bodice-ripping fast. Just quick fast. That's not to say couples can't have fun during the fast route. With the right company and CDs, even the express route can be all right. Still, you're clear on why you're there on this particular day of the month, involved in an encounter that has the spontaneity of a presidential inauguration. You're there to get the deed done, to get the conquering band of sperm to swim their way to the wooing egg.

During an extended time of such increased stress, many couples completely cut out the scenic route and get together only for fast trips. But that harms the relationship.

Because men generally enter intimacy through physical interaction, times of lovemaking that focus on love rather than on babies are especially important for a husband's emotional connection. Women tend to enter intimacy through verbal interaction, and a wife may overwhelm her man with the need to be heard but avoid sexual intimacy—the very act that helps him feel close to her. By making extra effort in each other's dominant area (usually the wife meeting sexual needs, the husband meeting verbal needs) couples can strengthen their marital health during these trying times.

As the window of fertility remains open only for a short time, the rest of the month provides ample opportunities for the slow and scenic, erotic and passionate. No man wants to think he's there only as a sperm donor, to provide genetic material for "the baby." He would much prefer to be the loving husband of a responsive, even aggressive, wife.

We encourage couples to ask each other, "Am I doing all I can to meet your physical needs?" and "Am I doing all I can to meet your relational needs?" Both are legitimate needs. (The workbook in appendix 1 has exercises that will help you with sexual intimacy.)

Sex and the Bible

We don't have to read very far in the Bible to find the subject of sex. It's implied in chapter one with the first command: "God blessed them, saying, 'Be fruitful and multiply'" (Gen. 1:22 NASB). That's a poetic way of telling the humans, "Make babies."

If we are to assume that "be fruitful and multiply" is a mandate that requires the faithful to pursue all means—expend all resources and use all technology, even cloning—to fulfill this command, it would seem that *everyone* must marry. Yet we know this is not so, from what we read in the New Testament (1 Cor. 7:8).

A few chapters after the first command in Genesis, we read about the first romantic encounter: "And Adam knew Eve his wife; and she conceived" (Gen. 4:1 KJV). More modern translations say that Adam "lay with" or "had relations with," but the older translations were closer to the original: "knew." Sexual intimacy at its foundation is about "knowing."

Fast-forward to Leviticus, where God instructed Israel to abstain from sex during the menses and for the seven days that followed. Some have wrongly suggested that this protracted period of abstinence made men more fertile, but semen quality actually diminishes after five or more days of abstinence, owing to the accumulation of dead sperm. (However, once ejaculation has occurred, good sperm quickly become available again.)

God's instructions moved the time of intercourse closer to midcycle, when fertility is actually enhanced. Thus, if God's chosen people followed his laws, they would have been directed toward a more fertile time of the cycle—and for women, thanks to hormones, generally a more pleasurable time (though modern medications can destroy that chemistry for infertile women). This was contrary to the "science" of the day. For centuries, it was believed that human females were fertile during the time of menses.[2] Yet the Bible strictly prohibited sex during the *presumed* fertile time.

The Old Testament includes additional times of abstinence, including the evening before worship and forty to eighty days after the birth of a child. Going back to these Old Testament dietary and ceremonial laws, however, negates the freedom of new covenant living. (See Acts 10:13–15, 1 Cor. 8:8, and 1 Tim. 4:3–4.)

If we flip forward to Song of Solomon, we find a book of the Bible devoted completely to marital sexual love, with no mention of children. It appears that in addition to God's plan that we populate the planet, he also intended sex for pleasure. In the New Testament, husbands and wives are exhorted to give themselves fully to each other, lest they be tempted because of too much abstinence (1 Cor. 7:5). This text also makes no mention of procreation, but implies instead a duty or responsibility for meeting each other's day-to-day sexual needs.

A survey of the church's view of sex through the centuries reveals that many leaders taught, "Whenever you have sex, conceiving babies must be a possibility." This is formally called the "unitive-procreative" link. The uniting act of intercourse was connected to the potential for procreation. Seeing an inseparable link here, some church leaders decreed it immoral for anything artificial to block the possibility of conception. Later a broadened interpretation was added to this guideline: nothing may artificially *prohibit* conception. This addition allowed pregnant and postmenopausal women—women who cannot conceive—to have sexual relations without violating the unitive-procreative principle because they weren't prohibiting conception.

Many early church leaders interpreted Scripture to emphasize family in terms of future generations, and they concluded that the primary goal of marriage was procreation. For many, eternal life meant having offspring that continued the family line forever. Reproduction was viewed as a link to eternity. Procreation was the most promising route to immortality, as men and women passed on their genes and their values and thus lived on. Interestingly, this immortality idea is the very argument used by some who advocate cloning for reproductive purposes.

Even more extreme was the belief held by some church fathers that the *only* purpose of marital sexual intimacy is reproduction. Many thought sex itself, even *with* the possibility of conception, was sinful; after all, would God want people to have *that* kind of fun, with all that gasping and sweating? They saw it only as a necessary evil for the continuance of the human race.

One leader stands out in contrast to this thinking. A third-century church father, Lactanius (ca. A.D. 250–325), appreciated the "joy of union," believing that the desire of a husband and wife for each other was God-given. He held that sexual expression within marriage had the added dimension of pleasure.[3] Yet the better-known Augustine, viewing intimacy through the grid of his own promiscuous preconversion state, emphasized the necessity of always, in each encounter, having a connection between intercourse and the possibility of conception.

While Lactanius held the minority view in his day, today most people of faith agree with him. While many preachers in the Renaissance said Christians should have sex only for procreation, and then only in the "missionary position," the prevailing view today is that lovemaking within the bonds of marriage is a good thing. Nevertheless, the unitive-procreative link as the purpose for marriage continues to pervade much of the church's thinking and influences many church teachings about reproductive technologies. (Such teachings include prohibition of contraceptives, manual sex, oral sex, donor insemination, and insemination using the husband's sperm.)

Couples today who hold to the unitive-procreative construct while pursuing infertility treatment sometimes engage in relations using specially designed, nonspermicidal condoms so that semen can later be removed and used for insemination. In such cases, condoms (i.e., birth control) are considered acceptable because their use is actually intended to aid procreation.

Procreation Only versus Pleasure and Procreation

Scholars of the past lacked the benefit we now have of knowing modern physiology, that wonderful science of studying God's design of mankind. They did the best they could without knowledge of the anatomical complexity and neurological diversity that cause sexual satisfaction for men *and* for women that has nothing to do with procreation. Here's some of what we now know.

How our bodies work. The female has a marvelous pleasure center: the clitoris. It has an enormous number of nerve endings, and unlike any other body part, male or female, its sole purpose is for sexual pleasure. In past centuries, little was known about the clitoris, perhaps because men could be sexually satisfied so quickly. Yet the very existence of a woman's clitoris suggests that God intended sex for pleasure.

Endorphins. Another unique design that links sex with pleasure but not with procreation is the phenomenon that happens in both men and women when orgasm occurs. After appropriate stimulation, the neural brain wiring causes explosive spasms of pleasure and the release of endorphins, powerful morphine-like chemicals.

Location of the clitoris. The location of the clitoris suggests that God designed sex for pleasure (see figure). More than half of women surveyed can't reach the endorphin surge without stimulation in addition to intercourse. The most definitive study on sex done to date demonstrates that approximately 67 percent of all sexually active women can't achieve orgasm via vaginal penetration alone. Even after altering positions and controlling the tempo of lovemaking, most women need more direct clitoral stimulation than vaginal penetration provides in order to experience an orgasm. In a study of Christian women, 59 percent said they were unable to have an orgasm during intercourse. Most who reach orgasm do so by stimulation of the clitoris with their own or their partner's hand, or by oral stimulation. Others use vibrators. A smaller percentage reported that they rely on external penal stimulation. All this is to say that if God intended sex only for making babies, we might expect to see the clitoris inside the vagina (though that would certainly add an extra challenge to childbirth!).

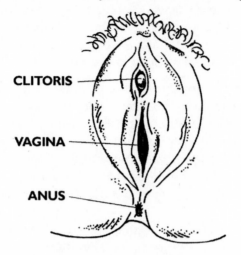

The sexual response cycle. The possibility of multiple orgasms in the female also suggests that our Creator designed us to enjoy sexual pleasure as well as to propagate the species.

And orgasm teaches us something about divine design. Men and women differ in the time they need between foreplay and orgasm. The average male can go from excitation to climax in three to five minutes. Yet in a study of 2,000 Christian women, 62 percent said they needed at least fifteen minutes of appropriate stimulation following arousal to reach orgasm. A small percentage said they needed more than forty-five minutes, and 1 percent needed an hour or more.[4] Such a difference in time requires communication and selflessness for both partners to be satisfied.

> *After reading some old Christian texts I came away with the idea that every time my husband and I came together, it had to end in intercourse. And not only that, I got the idea that I was less of a woman if I experienced orgasm in any way other than intercourse. As a result, every time I'd get "close," we would quickly move to intercourse. Sadly, each time I lost the needed stimulation, and I was left frustrated. This went on for ten years. I went from being multi-orgasmic to having a total of two orgasms in an entire decade.*

Now consider the impact of the "fast-trip-only" love lives of many infertile couples. When the wife is most fertile, both husband and wife may prefer the "three-minutes-to-mighty-sperm-eruption" sex. She chooses not to focus on her own physical needs because the baby quest is such a distraction. At first he may enjoy the "fast trip." But after a while, he may feel used. She isn't "getting together with him" because she desires him but because she wants something. He may then feel less inclined during the "off season" to want to invest the time it takes for her to experience orgasm. Yet that's exactly what's needed. A couple must make that "slow trip" a priority to keep their marriage healthy.

Female versus male approaches to sex. In general, women approach sex seeking the ultimate love experience, and men approach sex seeking the ultimate erotic sensation. A typical woman desires sex after she feels close to her husband; a typical man feels close to his wife after he has had sex with her. While verbal communication, more than a sexual encounter, may work as the initial door to intimacy for her, sex is still important and pleasurable for her and is a factor in her degree of marital satisfaction.

Secular humanists have long argued that the reason men are sexually satisfied so quickly is because of the evolutionary advantage. The rationale has been, "They had to get in and out fast because men were vulnerable to outside predators during the sex act." Why, then, have women persisted in the "slow mode"? Why do women have a sexual response at all? Why can women get pregnant without orgasm? Women's slower more relational approach suggests a Designer who intended an added dimension to sex beyond procreation: intimacy.[5]

It's Who You Know

The implications of viewing the purpose of marriage as being unitive-procreative versus "knowing" are enormous. Those focusing on "knowing" remind us that God is a relational being, and he created human beings for the purpose of relationship. For those blessed with a marriage relationship, we come to "know" our spouse intimately. This intimacy includes not only a physical relationship but also a spiritual and emotional connection.

White or wheat? Black or with sugar? Extrovert or introvert? Task-oriented or people-oriented? These are some initial questions to which one finds the answers in the first stage of "knowing" in a relationship. Then within marriage, there are the deeply intimate questions: "What are your erogenous zones?" "Do you like your kisses wet or dry?" "Do you prefer scantily clad or nude?"

The "knowing" model appreciates sexual expression within marriage as the joyful pathway to intimate knowledge as God designed. We encourage infertile couples focused on baby-making sex to focus on knowing each other. While the "fast trip," taking the highway or the speedboat, is completely devoid of bells, whistles, and fireworks, couples in treatment need the "pleasure cruise," the gondola ride or the scenic highway, for relational health. When couples can slow down and enjoy the scenery, they draw strength from their intimate times together, which can buffer them against the stresses of treatment.

While we may hold firmly to "knowing" as the main purpose of sexual intimacy, we respect and recognize the consistency of those who see an inseparable link between sex (the procreative act) and lovemaking (the unitive act). Before artificial insemination, couples had to have sex to reproduce. Since the development of ARTs (assisted reproductive technologies), couples must now decide whether they can legitimately separate the act of procreation from the unitive act of lovemaking. Those who see an inseparable unitive-procreative link thus view ARTs as unethical. Those who view the purpose of sex as "knowing" feel freer to use ARTs. For those who believe the latter, we'll consider some additional ethical issues in the chapters to follow.

Not *all* of the news about infertility and sex is depressing. Some couples who make physical expression a priority at times other than midcycle find renewed appreciation for what they can create together— a beautiful picture of oneness.

> *After all we've been through, having relations is a way of feeling protected, of making me feel desired and beloved. My husband takes so much care that sometimes when I moan with pleasure he stops to ask if I'm hurt.*

> *At first after we adopted, we thought our love life was suffering because of the leftover effects of infertility. Then we talked with couples who had newborns and we realized fertile couples, too, were experiencing similar challenges. Maybe it had more to do with being up in the middle of the night—we were tired! Today we like sex and rarely think about those high-pressured past encounters, so I guess you can recover.*

DISCUSSION QUESTIONS

For Couples Only

1. What are your erogenous zones? Do you like your kisses wet or dry? Do you prefer scantily clad or nude?
2. Ask each other, "Am I doing all I can to meet your physical needs?"
3. Ask, "Am I doing all I can to meet your relational needs?"
4. Are you happy with your love live? Why or why not?
5. Is the "slow trip" still a priority? Why or why not?
6. Has your love life deteriorated to the "fast trip" only? How can you change that?
7. What steps can you take to deepen the level of physical intimacy between you and your spouse?

For Couples or Group Discussion

1. Do you lean toward unitive-procreative or "knowing" as God's purpose for sexual intimacy? What is your religious background, and what are the ethical implications of ARTs in light of what you've been taught?
2. Which of these two constructs (unitive-procreative or "knowing") does your church hold to?
3. Can you, with a clear conscience, proceed with a practice that clearly violates the teaching of your church? What do you think of the ethics of masturbation to obtain a sample? Intrauterine insemination (IUI)? In vitro fertilization (IVF)?

For more on this subject, see appendix 1, which includes a section on sexual intimacy.

Chapter 9

THE MEDICAL WORKUP

COLLECT THE CLUES

*I finally worked up the nerve to see my ob-gyn because I hadn't con-
ceived after trying for more than a year. I was overdue for my Pap
smear anyway. Through the entire examination, I said nothing about
my fertility questions. Then the doctor, noting that we'd been married
five years, asked if we had given any thought to the "if or when" of having children. To the surprise of both of us, I burst into tears.*

*Being over thirty-five, I called the doctor after we'd been trying for six
months. I knew I didn't have time to mess around, and I had a thousand
questions. Were we infertile? If so, what was ahead? How much would
it cost? Would it hurt?*

Patients arrived at my (Dr. Bill's) ob-gyn office seeking help for a
variety of problems. Sometimes they stated the real issues; other times
I discovered their reasons during the history and the physical examination. Often a woman would arrive for her scheduled annual Pap
smear and, only as the visit was concluding, mention that she and her
husband had questions about conceiving. These timid, "by the way"
statements always sounded a warning.

Perhaps patients feared hearing, "Hmmm, it sounds like something's wrong," or worse, perhaps they thought I'd say, "It's all in your
head." Most patients have to muster up nerve to tell their doctors,
"We've been trying, but nothing's happening." Many cases begin with
patients in denial.

Some women did ask me for information before trying to conceive,
but most couples understand the basics of "makin' babies." So the topic
rarely arose unless they had already tried without success.

I generally took casual comments seriously, but I also knew that most women simply wanted reassurance—the doctor's blessing that all was well. After all, we had just concluded a thorough physical examination following a detailed exploration of complaints and family history. If I found nothing and pronounced her well, didn't that imply fertility?

Not necessarily. The annual physical or the routine examination with Pap smear is a screening evaluation for many chronic or acute diseases. The goal of this visit is to rule out conditions that we can successfully manage with early diagnosis and treatment. Thus, the annual exam is more about health and wellness than about the specifics of fertility.

Conception is a remarkably complex event involving female *and male* anatomy, physiology, and endocrinology. And though the husband may accompany his wife to her annual checkup, he certainly is not examined at that time. If the doctor is a known infertility specialist, couples are more likely to schedule infertility consultations and come in together.

Often the first clinician to perform an infertility workup is the ob-gyn. In fact, by the time patients have purchased a book about infertility, chances are they've already been through the initial medical examination. For the female, that includes a thyroid exam, assessment of hair distribution, a breast exam, and a pelvic exam. These examinations may provide clues as we look for unusual growths, infection, sores, or discharges. We also check cervical mucus for infection. We can find many subtle clues about hormone status through careful examination of the patient. And any suspicious findings prompt further evaluation of a given hormone level.

From here, while dependent on many components, the workup follows a logical progression that the patient can understand. Regardless of a patient's age when beginning a workup, the steps for diagnosis of infertility are the same for all. Yet for older women or women with histories of irregular periods and pelvic problems, we expedite the process because time is of the essence. It may take three or four cycles to complete the female workup because some tests must be done at specific times in the cycle.

The cost of an infertility workup can run several thousand dollars. More insurance companies cover the diagnostic workup than cover the treatment, as infertility can be a symptom of a variety of problems. I recommend that every couple at this stage seek to know the lingo and acquaint themselves with the available tests and procedures.

The information gleaned from the workup leads either to more tests or to a definitive treatment plan. All the while, we try to avoid jumping to conclusions based on small amounts of information. Otherwise the doctor-patient team can overlook important evidence and thus waste precious time.

Perhaps the simplest intervention involves education about the details of the human reproductive cycle. Husbands and wives who understand when the fertile period occurs can figure their optimal time for conception.

The History

Like a good detective, the diagnostician seeks clues and assembles them to guide his or her decision making. We start by getting a thorough history, which involves investigating the patient's health background. Some clinics obtain this information through an interview with the nurse or doctor, while others use a written form that the patient completes. Most clinics use a combination of both. All pertinent information becomes part of the chart, the permanent patient record.

Previous surgeries, infections, pregnancies, and allergies may all yield clues. We also investigate the menstrual history, past contraceptive use, current sexual patterns, significant health problems, lifestyle, and environment (especially exposure to toxins). Patients should bring to the initial visit pertinent information such as dates of surgeries and hospitalizations, medical records, and lists of any allergies they may have. They should also bring information about any medications they are taking or have taken in the past. As the mystery unfolds, this data may become more valuable over time.

A thorough history includes questions about a woman's family history of endometriosis (more on this later), hormonal problems, infertility, fibroids, and genetic abnormalities. It's also important to inform the medical team about any sexual exposure that might have resulted in a sexually transmitted disease (STD). Chlamydia and gonorrhea have enormous impact on fertility. Other common STDs such as herpes or HPV (human papillomavirus, or venereal warts) don't generally decrease fertility, but they affect the management of pregnancy once conception has occurred.

Besides the past history, the medical team will need to know what's happening now. Are menstrual cycles regular and predictable? Has the amount of flow or number of pads or tampons changed in the past year? Has there been any change in the intensity or character of cramps? Every woman is entitled to one irregular cycle per year, but when she can identify no recognizable pattern to her cycles, this is significant.

Does the husband or wife experience pain with intercourse? Is such pain new in location or character? Changes in bowel or bladder function may hint toward endometriosis or fibroid growth. Is there any new or unusual vaginal discharge? What are the couple's patterns, if any, of smoking and alcohol use?

The husband is asked questions about any problems that might be pertinent, such as infections, (STDs, mumps as a child), genetic disease, or infertile family members. This history, including medications past or present, provides clues that may add weight to one focus of the evaluation or alter the timeline for introducing more complicated, invasive procedures.

Examination of the Male

A critical initial clue in the examination of the male involves the availability and delivery of normal, healthy sperm. *The expert investigator will assess sperm through semenalysis early in the process.* Pursuing treatment of the wife without this simple assessment of the husband may cost the couple a lot of time and expense.

For decades, many people believed that if a man could achieve erection and ejaculation, infertility must be the woman's problem. But once we began to analyze semen, we found that fertility problems in men were as common as in women. And male infertility has been on the rise. In addition to aging, there are environmental factors. For instance, medications given to soldiers in the Gulf War have been linked to male infertility. Industrial solvents are also known to put fertility at risk.[1] Fortunately, in the last decade, we've seen particular progress in the treatment of male infertility, which had lagged behind treatment for female infertility.

Examination of the male can reveal undescended testicles or varicocele (British: varicocoele), an enlarged vein in the scrotum, which is the most common cause of male infertility. We also look for hair growth pattern in the genital area (hair pattern is a hormone-dependent phenomenon) and make a general examination of the penis and scrotum for abnormalities.

We had been trying to get pregnant for over a year before discovering that I had undescended testicles. Our doctor was surprised no one had ever diagnosed me. I am completely sterile. It was a huge shock.

I would hate to be a guy going through this. Even though I've endured more invasive procedures during the workup, my husband has to orgasm on demand. I couldn't do that.

When I went to give my specimen, I thought the doctor wanted urine, not semen. I called out through the door to the nurse to ask if I needed to fill the entire cup. When I heard her emphatic "No," I realized my mistake.

We had to reschedule the semenalysis a couple of times. I just couldn't perform under pressure.

In my practice, we encouraged the husband to obtain his semen specimen privately at home with his wife's assistance if they lived within an hour of the office. Then we'd have them bring the specimen in immediately, getting it to the office by 3 P.M. That way if the pressure of obtaining a specimen caused a delay, we had some flexibility in getting the specimen to the lab before it closed.

In one case, I had finished the examination and told the husband we would need to evaluate his sperm count and other factors related to male fertility. As my nurse handed him the sterile specimen cup, he left the exam room and stepped across the hallway to the patients' restroom. Minutes later he handed the cup back to my surprised nurse, who labeled the specimen for the lab as if everyone did it that way. Just for the record, most men find they are unable to focus sufficiently in a restroom in the middle of a medical office to get a specimen in that short amount of time.

A normal sperm count runs over 40 million, though many men with sperm counts over 20 million impregnate their wives without high-tech intervention, and men with more than 40 million sperm can have enzyme factors that render them infertile. In addition to assessing the sperm count, we also consider the sperm's volume, movement (motility), formation (morphology), white blood cells, abnormal clumping, and fructose.

A survey of 1,300 men and women found that half of them considered male fertility testing an embarrassing topic.[2] Recently we received a message through our website from a woman asking why men get so removed and angry when diagnosed with fertility problems. Not all men respond this way. Yet fertility is often ego defining, especially for men, most of whom connect it with virility and performance. Thus, a diagnosis of infertility often feels like a threat to their manhood. This is reflected in research indicating that infertile men report a 42 percent decrease in their level of sexual satisfaction.

The workup for men is generally less expensive and less invasive than for women. At first I resisted getting tested, but after I considered everything my wife had to go through—all the charting, poking, and blood tests—the least I could do was take my specimen to the lab.

It was crushing to find out I had a low sperm count. I'm trying not to withdraw, and I'm working to view this as "our" problem rather than just "my" problem. At the end of the road we may end up with a child we might not otherwise have had. When I keep that in mind, it's worth it.

In addition to feeling their privacy has been violated, some men also struggle with an ethical dilemma, as described by a pastor's wife:

One of the couples in our congregation went to the doctor for an initial infertility workup, and they were told that the husband would have to masturbate. A nurse handed the husband a stack of pornographic magazines and instructed him to get a sperm sample. It made them wonder if they can ethically pursue treatment. What do I tell them?

Many clinics have "collection rooms" equipped with pornographic literature and videos to assist the husband in obtaining a specimen by masturbation. Most Christians object to this process because of its association with lust.

Some Christians hold additional convictions that ejaculation apart from an act of marital intercourse is sinful. This position can be maintained within an entirely consistent and ethical construct. Yet that belief need not impede the workup. One patient writes of how she and her husband pursued their goal of having children while being sensitive to her husband's concerns:

My husband had a very strong conviction against masturbation, causing much frustration when the issues of sperm collection for tests or insemination were important. We resolved this by having our doctor prescribe a special sterile "fertility condom" or "condom for insemination," allowing us to collect through the act of loving intercourse.

As mentioned earlier, special, nonspermicidal condoms are available through a variety of sources. Couples can perforate these condoms with a pin if they feel it is important to allow the possibility of conception while obtaining the specimen for evaluation. Although latex is less than ideal, this method provides an alternative to obtaining a sample through masturbation. Researchers are now developing a home sperm-count kit that will allow men to learn on their own whether their sperm count is adequate for conception.

Certainly the husband can obtain sperm without resorting to pornography. Some wives go with their husbands into collection rooms to assist them. Or if his wife is not present, a husband can fill his mind with images of her, avoiding the lust issue. Other couples obtain the sample at home (ironically, a glass baby-food jar is ideal for transporting the sample) before whisking it off to the laboratory. It's important to keep the sample close to body temperature and to let the lab know what time the sperm was collected. Sperm specimens must be fresh on arrival at the laboratory, and thus advance arrangements must be made with the medical office.

Once the medical team has the results from the semenalysis, they proceed based on the findings. For the man with a prostate infection, a simple course of antibiotics could be all that's required. Other patients need hormonal therapies such as thyroid and testosterone. Low andro-gens (male hormones such as testosterone and DHEA-S) can affect sperm quality as well as libido. Antidepressants or beta-blockers can cause problems with ejaculation, erection, and libido, so stopping or changing medication may be the answer for others.

As part of doing sperm analysis, some clinics will require the post-coital test (PCT, also known as the Sims-Huhner test or Huhner's test). It assesses the interaction between the sperm and the cervical mucus. Timing this test is critical; it must be done within roughly twenty-four hours of ovulation and immediately after intercourse. Thus, couples "get together" and then rush to the doctor's office. Using a speculum, the clinician then takes a small amount of cervical mucus, places it on a slide under a microscope, and examines it for the number of viable, actively swimming sperm. Other significant findings include white cells, estrogen changes in mucus, quality of sperm, and the ability of the sperm to "swim" in mucus.

Some doctors swear by this test, while most patients swear at it. As one husband said, "It's pretty hard to make love when your wife expects a command performance." Another patient observed, "It's like donating your body to science while you're still alive." Sometimes wives arrive flushed, pheromones filling the air, with heartbeats still elevated. Hav-ing allowed no time to "enjoy the glow," they must exchange the "bed of delight" for the exam table, with the desperate hope that the test will be normal so they'll never have to go through that again! Some couples consider this test the ultimate molestation of their love life.

> There is no inner recess of me left unexplored. Sex used to be beautiful and very private. Now it's degraded and very public. Tell me, did I pass? Did I ovulate? Did I have sex at the right time as you instructed me?

> Ordinarily my husband was the instigator of sex. Now I felt I had to seduce him. We ended up fighting instead of making love.

Knowing that this test is difficult for couples, in my office we expected some late arrivals and some out-and-out "failures," and we allowed extra time or flexibility in rescheduling. While studies suggest that there's no absolute correlation between "passing" this test and the ability to conceive, the PCT still provides some clues, and any clue helps us to put together pieces that can solve the mystery.

If semenalysis reveals a problem with the male, we can move ahead to find the cause. Diagnostic surgery can uncover hidden causes of male infertility, and corrective surgery can often repair the problem. A varicocele can be corrected surgically. For others, the "ductwork" has failed to develop properly, preventing sperm from getting through. And some men, because of a missing enzyme, have sperm that congeals and doesn't liquefy like it should. Sperm wash with intrauterine insemination (IUI)—a procedure in which sperm are "washed" and then injected directly into the uterus—can correct this. Surgeons may also reverse vasectomies or repair structural damage.

Evaluation of the Female

Obviously, both sperm and egg are crucial. While we evaluate sperm for quality and quantity, we also evaluate the wife's ovulatory function. While semenalysis is relatively straightforward, proof of ovulation is far more complex, often requiring a variety of approaches. Each clinic may have its own preference for how they gather this information and the order in which it's assembled. The patient's age may influence pace, as well.

We evaluate basic female anatomy by examination and by sonography. We also test cervical mucus for white blood cells, which indicates the presence of infection. And we run cultures for chlamydia. If we identify problems, medical or surgical intervention may follow.

Many patients begin by recording the wife's early morning temperature on the time-honored BBT (basal body temperature) chart.[3] BBT charts, when reviewed at the end of unsuccessful cycles, can indicate the presence or absence of ovulation. Rather than helping the couple predict when to "get together," the BBT helps us know after the fact whether the woman is ovulating. While by no means precise, the BBT chart involves the woman in better understanding how her body functions and can add to the effectiveness of other tests and recommendations.

We had enough temperature charts to line a pet store full of bird cages before I found out that I didn't have to indicate "intercourse arrows" throughout the entire month. The doctor needed to know about sex only during my fertile time. It helped to understand why I was charting.

At one point we hit the stage of almost total abstinence. I put in an occasional X on the chart so the nurse wouldn't get the impression that something was wrong with our marriage.

For an accurate reading, you have to take your early morning temper-
ature before you get up. One Saturday I dropped the thermometer and
it rolled under the bed. Because I couldn't move too much, I had to
awaken my husband so he could crawl under there to get it for me. He
started the day in a lousy mood.

I've taken my temperature for so many months that when a friend asked
last week what the temperature was, I said, "This morning it was
97.7." She clarified that she was asking about the weather.

A woman's morning temperature, taken before arising, has a slight
upward shift following ovulation. A normal menstrual cycle will usually look biphasic in that the basal temperature runs low—perhaps 97.8
to 98.2 degrees—in the first part of the cycle (follicular phase) and then
rises about half a degree following ovulation (luteal phase).

Evidence suggests that the temperature rise parallels the release of
progesterone upon ovulation. Thus, when the ovary shifts to progesterone dominance, the temperature goes up. The addition of arrows on
the chart to show when intercourse happened helps couples determine
in retrospect whether relations occurred during the window of fertility.

Not all clinics use BBT charts. Some recommend ovulation test kits
instead.[4] Some clinics use midcycle sonograms, and others use a combination of these approaches. If a patient is being assessed by ultrasound, BBT charts are less important. Some women experience breast
tenderness and midcycle pelvic discomfort at ovulation time.

One of my patients had tried to conceive for nearly a year when she
presented for help. Her history revealed a significant amount of ovula-
tion pain each month. Because of the discomfort, she usually avoided
intercourse around that time. She was surprised to learn that was her
most fertile time.

Most women also notice a change in vaginal discharge around the
time of ovulation. This happens when the cervical mucus responds to
fluctuating hormones. As estrogen rises at midcycle in preparation for
ovulation, cervical mucus increases in amount and "slickness." If a
woman checks her vaginal discharge, she will notice an increase in
"wetness" or a slippery feel if she places a tiny amount of the mucus
between her thumb and forefinger. In a normal cycle, this clear, slippery
mucus indicates ovulation is imminent. (Patients with polycystic ovaries
always have such increased estrogen and slickness yet never ovulate.)

After the release of the egg, progesterone rises and the amount of
mucus decreases. It also becomes cloudy and sticky. By assessing
increased cervical mucus, many women can time intercourse to coincide

with the period of greatest fertility. Sperm can live for several days inside the female's body, so couples can rest assured that they don't have to "get together" at the exact moment of ovulation.

The BBT chart also indicates whether the temperature stays up after ovulation, as it should, and how many days ensue between ovulation and the onset of the period. These subtle findings can offer clues for treatment.

The ovulated egg lives in the fallopian tube and somehow woos sperm for approximately twelve to twenty-four hours. For years, researchers have asked how sperm can find their way from the uterus up the fallopian tubes to the egg. (In response, someone invariably tells the old joke about how 90 percent of the ejaculate remains in the vagina because men hate to ask for directions.) Yet now we have some clues as to how this happens. Using rabbits, researchers have found that sperm, like heat-seeking missiles, steer toward the egg using temperature sensors. Apparently the site where fertilization occurs is warmer than other sites in the female genital tract. Thus, it is theorized that sperm find their way to the "hot" egg. Similar studies using pigs have shown no such temperature difference, so no one knows whether human eggs give off heat. Other researchers have found that the egg sends a chemical message that sperm can sense when they get close enough.[5] Regardless of how the sperm find the egg, they can live up to seven days inside the female and are capable of fertilizing the egg during the first three or four days.

The clues about ovarian function represent considerable pieces of evidence for the medical team. Doctors may evaluate ovulation using different methods, some more invasive and precise than others. Yet the only absolute proof of ovulation is the harvest of eggs during in vitro fertilization, or pregnancy itself.

The workup generally progresses from simple and less expensive tests to more complex, surgically invasive tests. Think of the infertility investigation as a mystery for which the husband and wife each bring their own satchel of evidence, and with the assistance of the medical team, all try to solve the mystery. Not all patients need every available test. The results of each chosen test crystallizes the diagnosis. Some results will guide the team directly into therapy.

Observant patients can recognize subtle changes and alert the medical team, who then determine what laboratory tests to run. Symptoms such as changes in hair texture, feeling cold, weight gain without dietary change, and even constipation as a general change may point to a thyroid problem. This can also cause irregular periods. Even small hormonal abnormalities can have significant ramifications. For example, low thyroid levels (hypothyroidism) may negatively affect fertility even though the values fall close to normal. The various types of thyroid hormone may balance each other out, yet the ovulatory environment may still be inadequate. Blood tests provide the necessary evidence here. Thyroid problems are easily corrected.

Male hormones (androgens), which females also make in small quantities, can impact fertility, as well. If androgens are slightly elevated, fertility problems may result. Women with elevated androgens may notice oily skin, acne, hair growth in unusual places, and even changes in sex drive. Symptoms often develop over a long period and remain unnoticeable. Again, blood tests will reveal the levels, and if necessary, the patient may take oral steroids to normalize the androgens.

Prolactin, a hormone involved in the production and release of breast milk, is elevated in nursing mothers. Occasionally, however, a nonnursing woman attempting conception will have an elevated prolactin level. When sufficiently elevated, prolactin blocks ovulation and, in rare instances, can indicate a tiny tumor on the pituitary gland. The doctor will ordinarily check this hormone level, ask the patient if she has noticed a milky secretion from the nipple, and look for milky or bloody breast secretion. Oral medication can normalize this hormone level; only rarely do patients require more invasive procedures.

Discovering I had elevated prolactin seemed like the ultimate irony. I couldn't have a baby because my body thought I was breastfeeding!

Estrogen and progesterone receive most of the focus when it comes to female hormones. The ovary produces these hormones in a complex, synchronized fashion. When estrogen and/or progesterone levels are abnormal or out of sync, ovulation either fails to occur or it occurs in a way that inhibits conception. If we find that the wife is not ovulating, we check thyroid and blood-sugar levels. We use oral medications to treat thyroid problems and Glucophage to stabilize blood-sugar levels. At this point, assuming no complicating variables, we might start nonovulating patients on the low-tech ovulation inducer, clomiphene citrate (brand names: Clomid, Serophene, Milophene).

"Messenger hormones" called luteinizing hormone (LH) and follicle-stimulating hormone (FSH) regulate all female hormones. These messengers are secreted from the pituitary gland and tell the woman's body what hormones to produce throughout her cycle. The brain regulates the messenger hormones, and we assess them through blood tests. Abnormal production or exaggerated ratios warrant investigation and treatment. Also present in the male, these hormones are vital in the production of testosterone and maturing sperm. While estrogen and progesterone can be supplemented, most fertility treatments focus on stimulating ovulation by working with the messenger hormones.

After checking all hormone levels, if necessary, we can direct ovulation induction, which stimulates egg release. If it appears the patient is ovulating, we next look for evidence of endometriosis (more on this in the next chapter).

Effective treatment for infertility requires an accurate diagnosis followed by appropriate therapy. The male and female reproductive systems are highly complex and have the potential for many glitches. As each item in this short overview could be a chapter in itself, we encourage readers to consult with their medical team and to read the appendixes for additional sources of up-to-date, in-depth information.

In an infertility workup, the detective work must be methodical and complete before we can recommend appropriate treatment. Occasionally we can begin treatment plans while still doing further investigation. If the semen looks good and ovulation appears regular and precise yet conception still has not occurred, we move on to more invasive and expensive testing.

DISCUSSION QUESTIONS

1. While reading this chapter did you remember additional symptoms you need to tell your doctor about? If so, what are they?
2. What information did you leave out during the initial examination because you considered it unimportant?
3. How would you rate the exchange of information between you as a couple and your medical team? What changes are needed?
4. Are both you and your spouse committed to what's necessary to complete the fertility investigation? Why or why not?

Chapter 10

THE CONTINUING WORKUP

When April 15 rolls around every year, we reacquaint ourselves with "if-then progressions." Line twenty-three may say that if you spent more than $10,000 on medical expenses, then you skip to line thirty-nine. Line forty-one says if you have no dependents, then you go to line forty-seven. You rarely go from the first line to the hundredth in set numeric order. The order you follow depends on many variables.

The same is true of the infertility workup. You may not go straight from semenalysis to blood tests to fertility drugs. If the sperm test comes back normal, the medical team proceeds with testing the female. If tests show she has an abnormal thyroid level, there's no need to hand her a prescription for fertility drugs. Here we will sketch the "one to one hundred" progression, but realize that depending on what clues are found at each step, your individual treatment plan will follow a different course.

Common Diagnostic Procedures

In continuing the workup for the female, the medical team proceeds by doing several common diagnostic procedures. First we look for structural problems. If the patient appears to be ovulating, we might suspect some sort of blockage or uterine problem, especially if abnormal bleeding is present.

Hysterosalpingogram

A hysterosalpingogram (HSG) can confirm the presence of scarring inside the fallopian tubes or abnormalities in the uterine cavity. The procedure involves injecting dye through the vagina and cervix into the uterus. Once the uterine cavity fills with the dye, if the fallopian tubes are open, the fluid fills them and spills into the abdominal cavity. We then take several X-ray images, which may tell us if the tubes are blocked and, if so, where. We can also see if the uterine cavity is of abnormal shape and if polyps or fibroids are present. Depending on the findings, surgery may follow.

I had some abnormal bleeding, so my doctor's office scheduled me over at the hospital for a hysterosalpingogram. (I knew I was truly infertile when I learned to pronounce that word.) The procedure took less than twenty minutes, and it was uncomfortable, not painful. But I felt like a chicken on a rotisserie when they clamped something onto my cervix and then I had to turn over. Afterward the test showed that, while my tubes were open, my uterus was of abnormal shape, which explains why I keep miscarrying.

The HSG is generally done at a radiologist's office, an X-ray department at a hospital, or a diagnostic X-ray center. The patient usually isn't told the findings at the time of the test. A radiologist (and sometimes the infertility specialist) later reviews the films and calls the patient with the results. Because of tubal spasms, the HSG sometimes gives false information.

Some clinics are now using in-office transvaginal sonography (a sonogram done in the doctor's office using a vaginal probe) and injecting fluid into the uterus to get the same kind of information obtainable through the HSG.

Endometrial Biopsy

Another tool for diagnosing various uterine abnormalities is the endometrial biopsy. Through this test, we can evaluate the uterine tissue or lining, the endometrium (*endo* means "inside" and *metrium* means "muscle"). The endometrium or uterine lining grows monthly in response to increasing estrogen levels. Following ovulation, the hormone progesterone matures this tissue, making it lush and ready for the embryo to implant. In the absence of a pregnancy, the lining sloughs off as menstrual flow, and fresh tissue starts growing for the next cycle.

To evaluate the endometrium, the doctor inserts a flexible plastic endometrial suction catheter through the cervix into the uterus. A small piece of uterine tissue is then aspirated (a little suction is generated by an attached syringe) into the catheter and removed. Patient discomfort is often minimized with a numbing spray, as placement of the catheter can produce cramping. Patients can take ibuprofen with some food about an hour prior to the procedure. The entire process takes only a few minutes, and most patients tolerate it well.

The tissue is then sent to a pathologist who determines if the endometrium is "in phase," meaning the hormonal effects look appropriate for the stage of cycle. Abnormal findings are usually hormone related, generally associated with progesterone production. Unfortunately, the specimen is occasionally inadequate and must be repeated.

Transvaginal ultrasound, sometimes in conjunction with a biopsy, is also used to obtain clues about the patient's endometrial health. A relatively small group of patients have a thin endometrial lining, which impacts their fertility. The thickness of the endometrium can be measured by ultrasound and compared to the pathologist's findings regarding hormone effect.

Diagnosing Endometriosis

In ruling out anatomical problems, the physician looks for evidence of endometriosis, another common cause of infertility. When normal endometrial tissue is located in an abnormal place, the patient has a disease called endometriosis. About 5.5 million North American women have endometriosis, and 30 percent of them suffer from infertility.

With endometriosis, the endometrial tissue, which should be present only in the uterus, sometimes appears on the surface of the ovary, the pelvic organs, and even the intestines. In these places, the endometrial tissue can't slough off as in normal menses, so it stays, grows, and often sets up an inflammatory reaction. This reaction may cause scar tissue or adhesions (which is tissue sticking together where it shouldn't). Endometrial biopsy does not provide any clues about the presence of endometriosis, as the biopsy is done on tissue inside the uterus, and these implants are outside the uterus. Thus, diagnosis ordinarily requires laparoscopic surgery to determine if endometriosis is present and to assess the extent of disease and damage.

I told my boss that I might need some time off to treat endometriosis. He held up a palm and said, "I don't want to know! Just tell me if it's communicable."

Ever since age fourteen, I've had frequent abdominal pain. For years doctors told me that the pain was all in my head. One doctor said pain was a natural event for all women, and he suggested taking Tylenol. At age seventeen, I had my first diagnostic laparoscopy. The results showed that I had mild endometriosis that was removed with the laser. The pain subsided for a while but gradually came back. I've now had four laparoscopies. Now that I'm grown up and married, I'm back seeing the doctor—this time for infertility.

I never had any discomfort, but during my diagnostic laparoscopy, my doctor discovered that I had "medium" endometriosis. I thought people with that disease were supposed to have pain to warn them.

Depending on where the implants occur, endometriosis may cause debilitating pain. Yet about one-third of women with endometriosis have no symptoms. The disease develops over time; thus older women are more likely to have it. If a patient's mother or sister has had endometriosis, the patient's chances of having it increase sevenfold.

As if all the myths about infertility weren't bad enough, endometriosis sufferers face the additional misconception that it's the "career woman's disease," said to be brought on because they postponed having children. The truth is that 60 percent of women with endometriosis experience their first symptoms before age twenty-five, before fertility begins to decline.

The exact link between endometriosis and infertility remains controversial. In some cases, such as when the tubes scar shut, we can readily see how closed tubes would impair sperm from getting to their destination. Yet patients with minimal disease often have fertility problems, too. We don't know exactly why. Some believe renegade tissue causes inflammation, which makes the body summon "cleanup cells" that also attack sperm. Another theory is that endometriosis affects the inside of the fallopian tube. The tiny hairlike projections that line the inner tube appear to act differently when exposed to fluid from women with endometriosis than when exposed to fluid from women without the condition. This theory, for which there is some evidence, focuses on a chemical cause.[1] While we don't know exactly why women get endometriosis, we do know that they are much more likely to also suffer from rheumatoid arthritis, lupus, chronic fatigue syndrome, fibromyalgia, and allergies.[2]

Women with endometriosis often have menstrual pain that increases with age. They may also complain that a particular spot on their bodies hurts whenever they lift something, exercise, or have intercourse.

Infertility rates correlate with the severity of disease. Whatever the cause, treatment involves getting rid of the endometrial implants, either by surgery or with medication. Most specialists grade endometriosis (minimal, mild, moderate, severe) during laparoscopic surgery. Pregnancy rates generally improve following treatment.

In some women, the abnormal implants actually lie within the muscle of the uterus—a condition called adenomyosis. This condition often occurs along with classic endometriosis. A woman with adenomyosis may experience menstrual cramps that worsen over time. Her uterus tends to enlarge and may feel particularly tender during examination.

Some patients with mild or moderate endometriosis are candidates for medication. Generally, conception is impossible during this treatment. The treating physician will weigh the risks and benefits and decide the best approach for the individual case. If an infertility patient has significant symptoms of endometriosis, the medical team may decide to go straight to surgical intervention.

In vitro fertilization (IVF) has been found to be superior to intrauterine insemination (IUI) for treatment of patients with endometriosis, especially for those with severe (stage 4) disease.[3]

Diagnosing Polycystic Ovarian Syndrome

Another common cause of infertility is polycystic ovarian syndrome (PCOS), a hormone imbalance condition that affects ovulation as well as other body systems. It's the most common endocrine problem in all women of reproductive age, affecting between 5 to 10 percent of women during their childbearing years. Women with PCOS either don't ovulate or ovulate infrequently. They also have evidence of elevated male hormone, which may show itself in acne, facial hair, and/or elevated blood-test levels. A considerable number of women with PCOS are overweight.

Clomiphene citrate (more on this below) is an excellent drug for the treatment of PCOS. While a substantial number of PCOS patients will ovulate, only about 40 percent will conceive. Clinical trials are reporting that for ovulation induction associated with PCOS, metphormin (brand name: Glucophage) plus clomiphene citrate (Clomid hereafter) is more effective than Clomid alone. For the treatment of irregular periods associated with PCOS, Glucophage therapy may restore ovulation in most women, though they'll usually require about six months of such therapy before achieving ovulatory periods.

Diagnosing Immunological Problems

Reproductive immunology is a relatively new, controversial, and rapidly expanding subemphasis in the field of infertility. Immunological infertility may involve specific antibodies that are generated to oppose antigens in the sperm or in the developing embryo itself. The body's immune system generally protects against invading bacteria, viruses, and other threats to the normal balance. But some women make antibodies that attack not only their own tissue (autoimmune diseases) but also tissue containing the father's genetic material, such as sperm and embryo, which the woman's body recognizes as foreign and thus as a threat. Antibodies can destroy these foreign cells or can disrupt the blood supply to the embryo, resulting in recurrent pregnancy loss.

Specialists in immunological infertility have identified a number of categories of immune response that can harm a pregnancy. At this writing, the treatments for diagnosed immunological problems have demonstrated limited success. Current treatments include anticoagulant therapy (Heparin, aspirin) to prevent clotting of the tiny blood vessels critical to the early pregnancy, infusion (IV drip) of white blood cells from the father to desensitize the mother's immune system so it won't make antibodies against his genetic material, and intravenous gamma globulin therapy to coat the antigens, thus preventing the mother's immune system from being revved into action.[4] If her body mounts no immune response, a pregnancy can progress normally.

If your doctor suspects the possibility of immunological problems, blood tests will often supply the diagnosis. Most likely, samples of your blood, as well as your spouse's, will be sent to a special lab for testing. It may take weeks to get the results.

Ovulation Induction

If we find the male has healthy sperm but the female has irregular periods or is not ovulating, we usually start with ovulation medication. The first medication prescribed is Clomid. Although Clomid is a fertility drug, and thus a treatment, we use it sometimes as part of the workup process so we can assess how the patient will respond to it. Compared with other ovulation-inducing medications, Clomid is simple to take (orally rather than via injection), is relatively inexpensive, and doesn't require a prescription from an infertility specialist. It also has a good response rate. For many patients, Clomid overcomes simple problems; pregnancy results, and everyone's happy.

Last month I started my second round of the fertility drug Clomid. I did three months of it last fall, and now I'm on double the dosage—double the pleasure. Do you hear the music to the Wrigley's Doublemint Gum jingle? As my husband said, "Double the Clomid, double the witch." I can't figure out today if everyone in the world is a moron, or if it's just the meds talking.

On Clomid I don't feel crazy. I do get the hot flashes, though.

My doctor won't even refer me to a specialist for more testing until I do the second round of Clomid. Even the specialists often do two months of Clomid before trying anything else. These doctors are on the drug companies' payrolls.

I had an identity crisis. I had always prided myself in being emotionally stable, and I didn't know how to deal with the intensity of the emotion. You don't even understand why you're crying all the time. It still takes me by surprise. . . . the times when I think I'm so okay, and I talk to one person that just triggers it. It drives me nuts.

Clomid, an antiestrogen, tells the brain that the ovaries are goofing off, so it sends more messenger hormone (FSH) to the ovaries, telling them to produce more egg-containing follicles. Most women who respond to Clomid produce one or two mature follicles seven to ten days after the last tablet. It is advisable that a patient on Clomid (or any ovulation-inducing medicine) be followed with ultrasound to monitor the number of maturing follicles. This confirms that the medication and dosage are working and helps to avoid hyperstimulation, a condition (rare with Clomid) in which the ovaries overrespond, enlarge to a dangerous size, and put the woman's health at risk.

While people often associate multiple births with the more high-powered injectable fertility medications, sometimes Clomid is to blame. But multiple births are preventable through ultrasound monitoring of each new dosage. Excessive follicle production can be observed, and couples may be advised to avoid intercourse during a cycle in which numerous follicles are present.

Clomid has a long track record of effectiveness and safety. For 5 to 10 percent of patients using Clomid, we do see an increase in twin births, but high order multiples (four or more) is extremely rare.

While Clomid protocols can vary, most doctors begin a five-day course of the medication between days three and five of a woman's cycle, with day one marking the onset of menses. Patients take 50-milligram tablets daily for five days, with a maximum dosage of five pills per day. A woman will rarely ovulate on four or five pills daily if she didn't ovulate at three pills per day. Thus, if a woman is unresponsive to 150 milligrams per day for five days, we ordinarily reevaluate and take a fresh look at all the clues to find out why her ovaries are unresponsive.

Clomid can cause abnormalities in cervical mucus (rather than being clear, copious, slick, and stretchy, it may be whitish, less copious, and not as slick—making it less favorable for conception). Thus, it's good policy to evaluate the mucus at midcycle at least once while the patient is on the Clomid. In addition, women who have been on Clomid for many consecutive months may become somewhat resistant to it, and it may actually become counterproductive, inhibiting the ovulatory process. Thus, even if apparently ovulating, the patient who has been on Clomid for three to six months without a pregnancy needs reevaluation and perhaps a month off from the medication. One study has found that among women younger than forty-three, the maximum benefit of Clomid with intrauterine insemination (IUI) was reached after four attempts.[5]

Artificial Insemination

The order of tests and treatments in the infertility workup will vary depending on what clues the medical team gathers. For example, couples with a male-factor or cervical mucus problem might bypass ovulation-inducing medications and go straight to artificial insemination using the husband's sperm. Artificial insemination is simply the depositing of sperm in the vagina near the cervix or directly into the uterus (IUI) with the use of a syringe. IUI is often used in the process of therapeutic trials, especially for couples who have unexplained infertility.

> One advantage to cold, detached IUI is that it created a clear dichotomy in our love life. We could reserve intercourse for lovemaking. It was nice to associate sex with only love again.

> I hated trying to conceive when my husband was not even in the same zip code. He'd drop off his sample an hour before I got to the doctor's office, and I'd arrive after they'd washed the sperm. When my doctor was finished with the procedure, I quelled the urge to ask, "Was that good for you? Do you have a cigarette?" Sometimes it was hard not to be cynical.

> One Sunday morning we went straight to church from the doctor's office, following an IUI. When we got there, a friend asked, "Did you get it up?" We were stunned that he would ask something so crass until we realized he was talking about the Christmas tree we'd cut down the previous afternoon.

With IUI, a man provides a sperm sample. The sample is then centrifuged to concentrate the sperm into a pellet, resuspended in a special fluid medium, and centrifuged again. This procedure may be repeated a number of times, resulting in sperm that has been "spun and washed." The purpose of this process is to rid the specimen of any material that might hinder the sperm's progress or incite an infection in the uterus once it's injected. (Jokes abound about how the sperm is submitted to "wash and dry" and how difficult it is to hang each sperm on the line to dry.)

When a couple has intercourse, only a fraction of the number of sperm make it into the uterus. IUI increases that number. The washed sperm are placed in a catheter, which is threaded through the cervix. The sperm are then injected through it into the uterus. The procedure can be done in the doctor's office and takes only a few minutes, although the wife must lie down afterward for about fifteen minutes.

Couples time IUI to coincide with ovulation and schedule an appointment as closely as possible to the wife's most fertile time.

Following IUI, the patient may have light cramping and/or minimal spotting but may resume normal activities. Success rates depend on the number of mature follicles present (observable through sonography), with the highest pregnancy rates coming from those who have coupled IUI with ovulation-inducing medication.

Once again, we consider the if-then scenario. The physician may recommend Clomid with IUI before performing a laparoscopy. But if a patient has symptoms of endometriosis or fibroids, the physician may suggest going straight to surgical intervention.

Laparoscopy, Hysteroscopy, Fertiloscopy

The last stage of the infertility workup involves diagnostic laparoscopy. Gone are the days when telescopes looked only into space. Now surgeons can gaze into the inner regions using a tiny telescope—a laparoscope.

Laparoscopy provides direct images of the abdominal cavity, the ovaries, and the areas outside the fallopian tubes. Patients usually have lots of questions, such as, "What does the surgery involve?" "What can it tell us?" "What are the risks?" "Is it painful?" And the more dramatic patient asks, "Will I die?"

Laparoscopy is a common surgical procedure. Generally done on an outpatient basis, it takes between thirty minutes and several hours, depending on whether endometriosis is present and whether some other procedure such as hysteroscopy (through which we view the inside of the uterus) is to be done at the same time.

During laparoscopy, the surgeon inserts a needle in the patient's lower abdomen, and carbon dioxide gas is carefully injected, using an instrument that monitors the pressure. Simply stated, we put a bubble of gas into the abdomen. Normally, the abdominal organs are pushed up against each other, so without the gas bubble, the surgeon really couldn't see or do anything. The anesthesiologist will tip the patient head-down a bit so that the gas rises to the pelvis.

The laparoscope is thin enough to be inserted through a small incision (about a quarter of an inch) near the naval. The scope is equipped with a lens and a special attachment that transmits light through the tube. Through a second or third small incision at the area of the pubic hairline, the surgeon inserts additional instruments to move structures, pick them up, or stabilize them for further observation. When all this is in place, the surgeon meticulously evaluates every structure: uterus, tubes, ovaries, and the pelvic lining (peritoneum). The doctor is looking for evidence of infection, endometriosis, scarring from prior surgery, or even structural irregularities the patient may have had since birth.

In about half of diagnostic laparoscopies, the surgeon discovers abnormalities, most of which are correctable. When abnormalities are found, different options exist for handling them. If adhesions or endometrial implants are found, some physicians use lasers to vaporize them; other physicians prefer to excise them. Depending on the nature of the problem, electrocautery may be used in addition to lasers. Suspicious areas can be biopsied, and ovarian cysts can be removed or drained.

Occasionally the fallopian tubes are blocked, preventing the sperm and the egg from coming together. This can be confirmed by one of two simple tests, tubal irrigation or chromopertubation. Both tests involve injecting colored dye through the tubes to determine if they are open or blocked. If the tubes are open, fluid flows out the ends of the tubes into the abdomen.

The ovaries sometimes develop cysts, or fluid-filled sacs, which can be harmless, causing only mild pain. But some cysts cause infertility or menstrual disorders. If the cysts don't disappear after a short time, the doctor may want to perform a laparoscopy to find out what type they are, since some ovarian cysts may need to be surgically removed. Tumors of the uterus can also be examined by laparoscopy.

Laser equipment can be hooked up to the laparoscope, allowing abdominal surgery to be performed without having to make an incision large enough to insert the hands. The laser, or light beam, works by vaporizing water. Since soft tissues are 85 to 90 percent water, the laser evaporates tissue as well. Using the laser, surgeons can slash adhesions, cut fibroids from the uterus, vaporize mild to moderate endometriosis, open blocked fallopian tubes, and destroy cystic structures, assuming none of these is too large or inaccessible.

Laparoscopy is often combined with hysteroscopy—a procedure in which a tiny camera at the end of a tube allows a doctor to look inside a woman's uterus. Using the hysteroscope, the surgeon can see any irregular structures, polyps, fibroids, adhesions, or congenital oddities.

Laparoscopy is the final step in an infertility workup, and many physicians agree that the workup is incomplete without it.

A new investigative tool is the fertiloscope, which is a small needle-like scope that goes through the back wall of the vagina into the pelvic cavity. Slightly larger than a large-bore needle, a fertiloscope can be used in the doctor's office in conjunction with local anesthesia. Saline is injected into the pelvic cavity, allowing the operator to examine parts of the pelvis that fall naturally into view. If no adhesions are present, the doctor can see the back of the uterus, the ovaries, and sometimes even into the ends of the fallopian tubes. Fertiloscopy is still experimental, so its usefulness is yet to be determined.

At this point, it's important to note that while many doctors' offices may be equipped to do the initial battery of tests and evaluations, they may not be equipped to handle the IUI sperm wash or serial sonography. (Serial sonography is a series of sonograms done daily or every other day to monitor follicle maturation until ovulation or to determine when to induce ovulation with an injection of human chorionic gonadotropin, HCG.) Even fewer offices have a seven-day-a-week lab capacity. While most couples do not begin the initial investigation with an infertility specialist, if months go by without a pregnancy, the consideration about which type of doctor to see becomes more important. How does the couple know if they need an ob-gyn, a urologist, a fertility specialist, or a reproductive endocrinologist? Before moving on to discuss high-tech treatment, we'll explore how to choose and work with the third party in your love life: the doctor.

DISCUSSION QUESTIONS

1. After reading about these tests, which, if any, sound like they might benefit you? Why?
2. If you've had any of these tests, what has your experience been like?
3. Have you taken medications that you felt altered your personality? If so, how did they affect you?
4. Did any of the quotes in this chapter resonate with your experience? Why or why not?
5. The information provided here is a cursory overview. For up-to-date, in-depth information on any of these conditions, we recommend www.inciid.org.

Chapter 11

THE DOCTOR

THE THIRD PARTY IN A COUPLE'S LOVE LIFE

I've been seeing an ob-gyn for seventeen months, and I sometimes wonder whether his credentials are sufficient. As I investigate infertility for myself, I find information that he doesn't seem to know. My husband thinks I need to "trust the doctor," but our case may be beyond his training. How do I know?

This patient asks an important question, one that every patient should feel free to ask and investigate. There are a variety of reasons for seeking a second opinion or changing doctors. A patient may choose a physician with excellent credentials but then find the doctor-patient chemistry lacks an essential element. Or perhaps the ancillary staff frequently falls short. Or they are so good that the doctor lets them handle all the patient contact, so the patient never consults with the physician. A variety of legitimate problems can motivate a patient to look elsewhere.

Often all that's needed is a second opinion for a fresh look at the data. But many doctors who start the infertility workup lack the specialized training to give the couple the best chance of conceiving as diagnosis and treatment grow more complex. Knowing this, sometimes friends—especially other infertility patients—are quick to recommend changing doctors. Part of what may make a patient hesitate to switch doctors is the denial associated with infertility: "Surely our problem is not *that* serious." So making such recommendations is an art as well as a science.

"Many physicians say they are experts in infertility when they are not," says Theresa Venet Grant, cofounder and public information director for INCIID (InterNational Council on Infertility Information

Dissemination). How do you know the difference between a family doctor, an ob-gyn, a urologist, and a reproductive endocrinologist? And which of these is best for you?

Requirements for Various Specialties

The various infertility specialties have differing educational requirements. After college graduation, a student generally attends four additional years of medical school to receive the M.D. degree. Upon graduation, that student becomes a *physician*. To specialize in ob-gyn, the new doctor completes four additional years, with little emphasis on infertility. At this point, however, the doctor can legally hang on the door a plaque that says Ob-Gyn—Infertility Specialist.

The *ob-gyn* doctor then demonstrates proficiency by taking a written examination and may take the oral board examinations after two years' practice. These exams may even exclude infertility issues, as infertility is now a separate subspecialty in the field of ob-gyn. After passing, the physician becomes a *board-certified ob-gyn specialist*. Such physicians are generally well equipped to handle basic evaluations and to perform procedures such as Clomid therapy, IUI, and laparoscopic surgery.

To become a *urologist*, the medical school graduate must complete five years of specialty training that focuses on problems of the male and female urinary tracts and the male reproductive organs. Again, routine studies may place little emphasis on evaluation of infertile patients. For male-factor infertility, urologists with a subspecialty in andrology are the most qualified experts, having completed two-year fellowships and passed exams to become board certified in andrology.[1]

A *reproductive endocrinologist* (RE) is a subspecialist in ob-gyn with advanced training (a fellowship) in reproductive endocrinology and infertility. While the typical ob-gyn resident receives between five and twelve weeks of training focused on infertility, a fellow spends two to three years in the field after completion of the residency. RE fellows are trained in advanced procedures such as difficult surgeries, tubal ligation reversals, and difficult laparoscopic surgeries. They also receive advanced training in the use of injectable fertility drugs (e.g., Pergonal, Follistim, Repronex) and in assisted reproduction procedures (e.g., IUI, IVF, and GIFT). Following a year of research and after publishing in a fertility medical journal, the subspecialist becomes "board eligible" in infertility. Then comes a written test and an oral examination to become a board-certified subspecialist in the field of reproductive endocrinology and infertility. Generally, we see these highly specialized physicians heading IVF clinics. Many of them accept patients only by referral following the infertility workup.

As you can see, there is an enormous difference in training between an ob-gyn "infertility specialist" and a board-eligible or board-certified reproductive endocrinologist.

Many patients, such as those in rural areas, do not have access to REs. Consumer groups recommend that after completion of the initial workup, if patients cannot find such a highly specialized physician, they should try to find a doctor who devotes at least 30 percent of his or her practice to treating infertility.

The director of a reputable IVF clinic suggests that some ob-gyns understand and can evaluate infertility well; some cannot. Because their jobs involve working with women, most ob-gyns know far less about male infertility. He suggests, "If you have been with a physician six to twelve months without a diagnosis or a pregnancy, it seems reasonable to pursue another opinion." It is always reasonable to pursue a second opinion and to ask your doctor whether his or her office is the best place to handle your case.

Once you find a doctor whose qualifications meet your needs, ask the name of the contact person at that office. Sometimes patients insist on speaking only with the physician, when highly trained staff members can handle many questions and are more accessible. Call the contact person to discuss any concerns, follow up on lab results, recheck dates, and confirm appointments. Labs can make mistakes, reports can and do get misplaced or misfiled, and crucial dates can pass unnoticed. These errors are somewhat rare, but the treatment process holds enough pain without added feelings of neglect or unnecessary fear.

Last time I saw my ob-gyn, he said he was going to refer me to a specialist. This time he seems to have forgotten that he said that. The past three times I've seen him, he wondered aloud, "Now, have we already checked your husband?" Each time I remind him that we have and what the results were. Why can't he seem to remember important information?

My doctor left me on bed rest with hyperstimulated ovaries and then forgot about me! Later he apologized, but not until I'd missed a couple extra days off work at a job that pays by the actual number of hours worked. I know mistakes happen, but it's hard not to be a little bitter. I'm just one of many patients to him, but treatment is just about my whole life.

An informed patient can be a tremendous asset and can add greatly to the efficiency of the evaluation and even to the success of therapy. No one knows your body or symptoms like you do, and no one will keep records as meticulously as you can.

Physicians' offices and infertility clinics can be busy, impersonal-feeling places. While most professionals involved in this specialty truly desire successful outcomes, tracking the vast array of lab results and cycle days can be challenging. So become informed and freely ask questions so that you can understand the plan and procedures.

It used to offend me when my doctor couldn't recall my case without looking at my chart. After all, I hung on every word he said, ruminating on our entire conversation until the next visit. How could he forget me so easily? Then I started working at a job where I interviewed hundreds of people in a week. I saw how hard it would be to keep track of so many names and situations without consulting my notes.

I overheard a patient reaming out the doctor for planning to be out of town during the time she would ovulate. He said his partner would be there to take care of her needs, but she didn't seem to care. The irony of it was that he was leaving town to attend a professional medical meeting!

Researching infertility information gives many patients a sense of empowerment, and they will read with only themselves in mind, which the doctor could never do. This can lead to good questions and reporting important symptom changes, which assists the physician in making effective adaptations in the treatment approach. Patients must recognize, however, that not all advice from books, friends, or the internet are actually pertinent to their particular circumstances. Medical journals are much more up-to-date than most popular publications, so keep a questioning tone rather than an insistent tone with your medical team. The well-qualified team examining you and evaluating your laboratory values is usually the best source of medical information. Learning to evaluate and apply data from reputable medical journals requires considerable training; attempting to make an accurate diagnosis using information from an anonymous person writing for a magazine is sheer folly.

While it's appropriate for patients to have high expectations from the person whose monthly Jaguar payment they're convinced they're financing, it's also important to have realistic expectations about what any one physician can do. Doctor-patient relations often improve when both the husband and the wife make it a priority to see the doctor together. Two sets of ears may hear the same conversation differently, usually with improved results. Patients have the responsibility to take care of themselves, to seek care when they have problems, to keep the doctor informed of any symptoms, and to follow the prescribed treatment plan. The husband and wife are ultimately the managers of their own care.

As questions arise throughout the month, jot them down and bring the list with you. Just keep in mind that writing a four-page, single-spaced list with questions in random order and "just dropping by to talk" will make your doctor want to head the other way whenever you show up. Ask your doctor the questions that are of highest priority to you.

Save the remaining questions for a call to the nurse or schedule a consultation-only appointment. At such an appointment, you don't have to undress and sit on a table, you don't have any tests done, and you don't endure any procedures. Instead, it's your time to ask the physician to review your treatment plan and answer your many questions. While there is a fee associated with such a visit, it's worth it to have your questions and concerns addressed without the anxiety of pending procedures or invasive tests. Some patients have found it helpful to schedule such an appointment every few months.

Patients also have rights. At present, there is no official, enforceable law detailing patients' rights. But you can certainly "vote with your feet" by taking your business elsewhere if you receive substandard care.

What are some of your rights? You have the right to respectful care. You have the right to receive information about your treatment and prognosis. You have the right to refuse a plan of care and to expect your case to be handled with confidentiality. And you have the right to know what your treatment choices will cost before the bill arrives. You also have a right to review and make copies of your medical records.

My doctor prescribed progesterone. When I read the packaging that came with it, it terrified me. "Deformities in offspring" was one of the possible side effects. Another infertility patient suggested I should get a new doctor. As it turned out, the packaging was warning about synthetic progesterone, and my doctor, having prescribed natural progesterone, knew it was perfectly safe. A more thorough physician would have warned me. But it wasn't worth leaving over it.

I received some anti-IVF literature that said 70 percent of all embryos die during the process of IVF. The author had taken the average 30 percent success rate and—failing to factor in cycles in which no fertilization occurred—assumed that meant a 70 percent embryo death rate. There's a lot of faulty information out there.

Improving Fertility without Medicine

Questions may well arise from what you hear or read, and it is perfectly appropriate to bring your questions to the medical team for clarification. Yet you can take some steps on your own to enhance your fertility. The following questions and answers may help you to do just that.

Should I change my diet?

Every month when I start my period, I think of all those chocolate bars and Pepsis that I gave up for . . . what? Nothing. It seems like such a waste.

Eating well will always contribute to your body's overall health. If your body fat is either too high or too low, making adjustments may enhance your fertility.[2] Also, caffeine affects fertility. Studies differ about how much has a detrimental effect—whether patients can consume two cups of coffee per day or if they need to limit themselves to one—but certainly three or four cups are too much if you're trying to conceive. Remember that chocolate, cocoa, some soft drinks, and black and green tea contain caffeine. Scientists in Denmark found that pregnant women who drank eight or more cups of coffee a day ran more than twice the risk of stillbirth compared with women who abstained from drinking coffee.[3] Women attempting to conceive should also limit their intake of tuna.

Women who drink alcohol should stop. Even moderate drinkers have lower fertility rates than do women who abstain.

Do health foods enhance fertility? Some over-the-counter herbs may actually decrease fertility for both men and women who take them. Researchers have found that high doses of echinacea, ginkgo, and St. John's Wort, in particular, impaired the ability of the sperm to penetrate the egg and also seemed to cause genetic mutations in the sperm.[4] The researchers did use hamster eggs rather than human eggs, and animal data doesn't always connect with humans. The study had several other flaws too. Nevertheless, just because something comes from a health-food store does not mean it's good for us. Due to quality control issues, many doctors hesitate to recommend or support using homeopathic remedies before they have been thoroughly studied. The exact contents of such remedies can be a complete mystery, and some ingredients can be bad for your health.

Still, if low fertility is linked to hormonal imbalance or nutritional deficiencies, nutritional supplements could play an important role in treatment. Research is currently under way, particularly with folic acid; vitamins E, B6, and B12; iron; magnesium; zinc; L-arginine; chasteberry; green tea; and selenium, to determine exactly what ingredient or combination of ingredients may be best for enhancing fertility.

Should I take vitamins? A good multivitamin will supplement your diet but should not replace healthy eating habits. Be sure to get a vitamin that *does not* exceed 5,000 international units of vitamin A but *does* include both folic acid and vitamin B12. Higher blood levels of folic acid in pregnant women may lower the risk of miscarriage. Women are advised to take folic acid supplements before and during pregnancy to prevent birth defects.

Warning: proceed with caution when you encounter any vitamin-selling company that claims a link between their product and improved fertility.

> *My whole lifestyle changed when I entered infertility treatment. I started eating totally healthy, taking vitamins, no soda, caffeine, junk, no carrying heavy things, no cleaning solutions, no more cleaning the cat box, no more electric blanket. You name it, I did it. I wanted to do everything I possibly could to be healthy.*

Do zinc supplements improve fertility? Zinc was used in the past to treat some types of infertility, and though zinc may not always work, it may help some men.[5] Reliable data is lacking, but a multivitamin containing zinc—not megadoses of zinc—may hold some advantages. Typically, as lead levels in the blood rise, zinc levels drop. And lead exposure may cause some cases of unexplained male infertility by impairing sperm. Men with high levels of lead may lower those levels by taking zinc supplements. Lead exposure can happen through contact with lead pipes, paints, ceramic glazes, pewter, and some types of metal utensils. In addition to lead, other environmental hazards such as exposure to pesticides and steroids should be avoided. And check with your doctor about any medications you are taking.

Are there other environmental factors I should avoid? When eating out, consider ordering something other than shark, marlin, and swordfish. A team of researchers found that 35 percent of women with unexplained infertility and nearly 40 percent of men whose semenalysis showed abnormalities had higher blood levels of mercury than did their fertile counterparts. They also found that both men and women with the highest blood levels of mercury ate the most seafood.[6]

A widely used industrial and household solvent has been linked to male infertility by a team of Canadian and U.S. researchers. The researchers suspect that trichloroethylene (TCE), a solvent used in industry to clean metals (car mechanics use it to strip grease) and frequently found in such consumer products as paint thinners, spot removers, and carpet-cleaning fluids, concentrates in the male reproductive system, where it impedes the growth of healthy and viable sperm.[7]

Perfume can also contain toxins. Thirty-four toiletries were found to contain phthalates, which enhance the ability of perfume fragrances to linger. Cosmetics that use the most potent forms of phthalates have been banned in some places out of concern that they cause genital abnormalities in up to 4 percent of male babies. Scientists believe the phthalates can be absorbed into women's bloodstreams through the skin or inhalation.[8]

Can exercise be harmful? You need to get proper exercise, but some women who exercise too much have light or nonexistent periods and fail to ovulate. Women in treatment should exercise moderately. Men appear to tolerate more exercise without negative results than do women. Men who like biking, however, should take note. An increasing number of studies link mountain biking and long-distance biking with decreased fertility. The same is true for long-distance truck driving. For men, the exercise-infertility connection relates mostly to elevated testicular temperature. And sitting for long periods makes the prostate more vulnerable to infection. The physical stress of bike racing also comes into play here. In one study using ultrasound, 88 percent of cyclists had abnormalities of the scrotum, including cysts, calcifications, and varicose veins. Compare that with about 25 percent of the control group.

What about smoking? In addition to having a negative effect on your health in general, smoking tobacco also increases a woman's risk of infertility. The effects of smoking and secondhand smoke on male fertility are less clear, but evidence points to it affecting male fertility as well. And marijuana smoking, whether by men or women, has a negative impact on fertility.[9]

Will using a hot tub hurt my sperm count? Anytime you raise the temperature of the testicles for extended periods, you have an increased risk of infertility, as the heat changes the process of sperm formation. Avoid long, hot showers and frequent use of hot tubs and saunas. It may help to wear boxer shorts rather than briefs or spandex shorts. Do not expect instant results, however, because the process of sperm production takes several months.

Does the pill cause infertility? There appears to be no connection between fertility problems and oral contraceptives used for any length of time. In fact, pill users have a reduced incidence of ectopic (tubal) pregnancy—which can be life threatening—as well as a reduced incidence of ovarian and uterine cancers.[10]

Is it possible to have sex too often—when trying to conceive, that is? At the time of ovulation, having sex every thirty-six hours is the general recommendation. More frequent intercourse may reduce the number of healthy sperm. A robust sperm count that is slightly lowered because of frequent intercourse generally presents no problem. But if the husband's sperm count is about 20 million and daily sex drops that to 15 million, there may be cause for legitimate concern.

Some couples avoid relations during the first two weeks of the cycle to "save up" more sperm. But since sperm die after several days, this practice actually reduces the number of healthy sperm in each sample.

At other times of the month, the frequency of relations has no effect on fertility.

Do both of us have to orgasm for conception to occur? No. In normal conception, only the husband has to orgasm for conception to occur. Ejaculation is vital for fertilization, but many babies have been conceived in the absence of female orgasm.

Do lubricants hurt our chances of conceiving? Perhaps. So avoid lubricants and douches during fertile times. Lubricants may hinder the sperm's ability to swim up the female reproductive tract.

Is it true that vasectomy reversals are rarely successful? No. With the advent of microscopic surgery, the statistics on vasectomy reversal are fairly encouraging. A report from the Johns Hopkins Medical Institutions suggested that patients have a better than fifty-fifty chance of fathering a child after vasectomy reversal. People who've had sterilization procedures followed by life circumstances such as divorce or the death of a spouse sometimes find themselves wanting to expand their families. However, the longer a man waits to have the reversal, the lower his odds that the procedure will work.[11]

Is there a scientific link between fertility and prayer? It would appear so. Researchers in one study discovered that women at an IVF clinic had higher pregnancy rates when, unknown to the patients, total strangers prayed for their success.[12] In the study, researchers found that of the 199 women involved, those who were prayed for became pregnant twice as often as those who were not the focus of prayer. The researchers said they initially hesitated to report their findings but ultimately decided the information was too significant to suppress. None of the patients knew about the study, nor did the medical staff caring for them.

While the data is too preliminary for us to be dogmatic, it certainly supports asking your friends, family, and church members to pray for you. And, of course, continue to pray for yourself. It not only deepens your relationship with God; it has the added benefit of improving brain health and function.

Working with Insurance Companies

One facet of working with the medical team is handling insurance issues. Learning all you can about your insurance options may save you a lot of money.

Before seeking medical help we learned that our insurance policy covered diagnosis but not treatment of infertility. Because we were at the diagnostic stage, we assumed they would cover us, so my husband went to the urologist. The diagnosis code assigned was "infertility," which we didn't know until the bills rolled in. Yet my husband had an underlying medical condition that was causing the infertility. After we had paid more than $2,000, the doctor made a final diagnosis: "Obstruction—male genital disease." If I had been more proactive in the beginning, we probably wouldn't have had to pay all that money.

According to the National Center for Health Statistics (NCHS), approximately 5.4 million couples experience infertility each year. Of those, fewer than 2 million seek help from the medical community. Yet if you're among those 2 million who seek help, you're going to rack up some medical bills.

The pain of treatment is bad enough, and then the financial stresses begin to mount. No federal law requires insurance coverage for infertility treatment. At the time of this writing, however, fifteen states require health plans to provide some sort of infertility benefits. Some states require coverage only for IVF; others require coverage of diagnosis but specifically exclude IVF. Sources such as RESOLVE (www.resolve .org) and the InterNational Council on Infertility Information Dissemination (www.inciid.com) provide insurance advocacy information.

My insurer initially refused to pay for some of my blood tests because infertility wasn't covered. When we told them we were trying to rule out thyroid problems—which is the truth—they reversed their decision and wrote a check.

If I can save a buck, I'm all over it. I've felt so helpless as I've watched my wife cry every month. Now handling the insurance battles is something I can do.

I represented a woman who had a laparoscopy because of pelvic pain. The insurance carrier denied the claim stating it was for the treatment of infertility. By taking the claim through the grievance process, eventually the insurance company paid benefits. We were able to establish that the laparoscopy was not done for infertility but for pelvic pain. More importantly, the contract only excluded "treatment" of infertility. Since the procedure was diagnostic, the insurance carrier determined that it was required to make the payment.

My insurance plan labels infertility "elective," lumping it in the same category as tummy tucks. I think it's especially sad that they'll cover abortion but not infertility.

In working with the doctor's office and with insurance companies, you, the consumer, have rights. And with rights come responsibilities. Stay informed so you can manage your own care. Be honest in all your dealings. You may not have as much control as you would like over your infertility, but you do have some control over getting the best care possible. Taking charge of your fertility will help reduce some of the feelings of helplessness that accompany the oh-so-stressful treatment process.

It's also important to have realistic expectations, a particularly difficult challenge when so much is at stake. As one patient wrote, "I want my doctor to be young enough to have all the new training but old enough to have lots of experience. I want him always to be available, yet I expect him to be balanced enough to take his family on vacation— as long as that vacation doesn't fall during the middle of my cycle. I'd sure hate to be my doctor!" How appropriate is the prayer of King David: "May integrity and uprightness protect me, because *my hope is in you*" (Ps. 25:21, italics ours).

DISCUSSION QUESTIONS

1. What are your doctor's credentials?
2. What does your insurance cover, and what's excluded?
3. Have you or your spouse felt your doctor was unqualified or incompetent to handle your case? If so, how?
4. Do you have confidence in the care being rendered? If not, why not? If so, why?
5. Have you sought a second opinion? On the basis of what you've just read, is a second opinion warranted? Why or why not?
6. What questions do you have for your doctor? Do you need to set up a consultation-only appointment?
7. What do you expect from your medical team? Are your expectations reasonable?
8. Do you usually take an active or passive role in your treatment? Why? Would your spouse answer this question the same way you did?
9. Do you need to take steps to improve your overall health? If so, what are they?

Chapter 12

State of the ARTs

High-Tech Treatment

~~~~~~~

Most couples who reach the point of using assisted reproductive technologies do so having already faced the foothills of damaged love lives, emotional upheaval, and spiritual crises. Now they must face the Mount Everest of financial, relational, social, spiritual, and ethical dilemmas that accompany these high-tech treatment technologies. At this point in treatment, nearly all of life gets screened through the perspective of infertility treatment. One patient complained that when her neighbor came over to ask if she had any eggs, she was offended until the neighbor clarified, "I meant *chicken* eggs."

After a couple has endured the infertility workup and perhaps has been in treatment for months, if not years, and they still have no viable pregnancy, the doctor may recommend high-tech treatment options known as assisted reproductive technologies—ARTs. We have already discussed intrauterine insemination (IUI), one such technology. Now we will move to the next level of options that include injectable medications and the various forms of in vitro fertilization (IVF).

The "Big Guns"

About 40 percent of infertility patients suffer from ovulatory problems. The ovulation process begins with the pituitary gland—located at the base of the brain, directly above the back of the throat—which produces hormones that stimulate the ovary (see fig. 1). The hypothalamus, a part of the brain that regulates the pituitary—tells the pituitary to release two pertinent hormones: luteinizing hormone (LH) and follicle-stimulating hormone (FSH), also called gonadotropins. These hormones signal the egg to develop in the ovary, an event accompanied by increased estrogen levels in the blood.

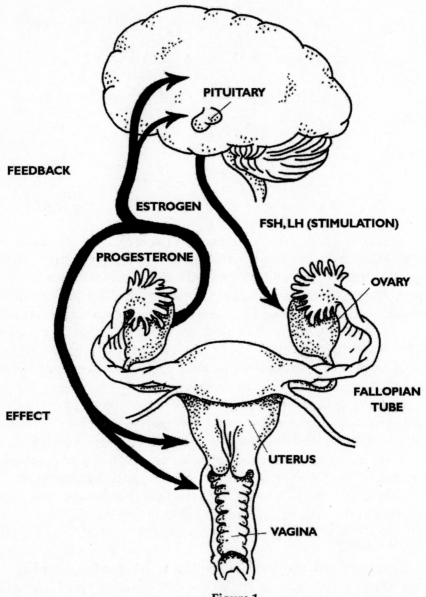

FEEDBACK

ESTROGEN

PROGESTERONE

PITUITARY

FSH, LH (STIMULATION)

OVARY

FALLOPIAN TUBE

EFFECT

UTERUS

VAGINA

Figure 1

Though the egg is microscopic, it grows within a follicle that we can see and measure with a transvaginal ultrasound (see fig. 2). Patients can recognize the follicle as a black circle on the screen. They often ask, "Is *that* normal?" and in fact, it's both normal and essential.

When the egg develops fully and the estrogen reaches a critical point, a boost of LH, one of the two key hormone messengers, signals the follicle to release the egg. That "releasing" event is ovulation. The egg then travels from the ovary and, assuming a fallopian tube is functional, is picked up or sticks to the delicate fingers (fimbria) that sweep the egg down the open passageway of the tube. The empty follicle that held the egg then begins to make progesterone, the hormone needed to support a pregnancy. If no pregnancy occurs, the progesterone level falls, causing the period to start.

Ovulation induction involves using a series of hormones to mimic the natural process of stimulating the ovaries to produce a ripened egg(s) that can then be fertilized. Both those with absent or irregular ovulation and those with unexplained infertility are candidates for an aggressive treatment approach to bring about ovulation.

The doctor may begin with a low-tech option: Clomid. If that doesn't work, it's time for the "big guns": the injectable ovulation-inducing medications, sometimes referred to as "the injectables."

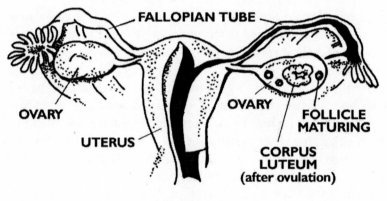

Figure 2

Bankruptcy by Injection

While a normal ovulation cycle requires the finely tuned release of precise amounts of FSH and LH, pharmaceutical companies have purified and synthesized these hormonal messengers into injectable form.[1] These medications originally required intramuscular injection (big needle, deep shot); now they can be given subcutaneously (small needle, shallow shot).

Ovulation inducers can be used in a variety of approaches. The hyperstimulation approach using gonadotropins (LH, FSH) can be used alone, along with IUI, or as part of the "recipe" for assisted reproductive technologies such as IVF. Using these medications, doctors can directly stimulate the ovary as though the pituitary didn't exist.

This powerful, expensive approach must be undertaken with great care.[2] With normal ovulation, the body has mechanisms that turn off the pituitary when enough messenger hormone (LH, FSH) is secreted. Yet when we bypass these safety valves by directly injecting the hormones, we must avoid potential complications through close follow-up of blood hormone levels along with ultrasound monitoring. A patient on these medications can develop ten, twenty, or more eggs that reach maturity in a single cycle.

A number of products contain either FSH and LH or pure FSH. Each medical team has its own preferences for what to use when, so defer to what your physician thinks is best in your case.

The injectables are generally given daily over a prescribed period of the cycle. For convenience, many patients give themselves the shots, have their husbands do them, or find a nurse or friend who's willing to help. The medical team watches the follicles develop, using serial ultrasound alone or in conjunction with blood estrogen levels.

The medical team can adjust the dosage of FSH/LH daily so that an optimal number of follicles reach maturity. Once the cysts containing the eggs are of appropriate size (and/or estrogen reaches the appropriate level), the patient receives a shot mimicking the natural LH surge to trigger ovulation. Ovulation generally happens within twenty-four to thirty-six hours. Most clinics use HCG (human chorionic gonadotropin) for this shot. It may be helpful to know that this hormone is identical to the one checked for when testing for pregnancy, so if you take a home pregnancy test at this point and for some time afterward, it will be positive. This does not mean you are pregnant!

Following the shot, patients receive specific instructions about the timing of intercourse or IUI.

My wife and I joke about the most awkward places where we've "done it." No—I don't mean where we've "gotten together" sexually. I mean where I've given her the daily hormone injection. To date the most cramped site was the bathroom of an airplane.

When I started in treatment for secondary infertility, my doctor prescribed Clomid. When that didn't work, I moved up to Pergonal and then Metrodin. It felt strange to worry that I'd never have another child while also fearing I'd end up with six in one pregnancy. Treatment involved daily shots in addition to sonograms and blood tests. It created scheduling nightmares for me at work. Fortunately, insurance covered a lot of it. Otherwise, it would have cost us several thousand dollars a month.

Counting the Cost of Injectables

Couples typically consider two key factors when they count the cost of injectables. The first is the monetary cost, and the second is the potential cancer risk.

I have friends who have been unable to do treatment because of money, and it's heartbreaking. High-tech treatment has been relegated to the better off and people with insurance. It's unfair that someone can't do treatment just because they can't afford it.

Cost. Some patients have found lower-priced, quality medications through reputable U.S. online pharmacies. The National Association of Boards of Pharmacy verifies the licensure of online pharmacies through their VIPPS (Verified Internet Pharmacy Practice Sites) program, so look for their endorsement at any online pharmacy you're considering.

A number of businesses offer low-cost loans for couples in treatment.[3] In addition, fertility medication manufacturers occasionally offer assistance for couples with limited incomes.

If the cost of ovulation induction alone is high, the cost of IVF is enormous. The median cost per IVF cycle is close to $10,000. Patients, on average, pay an estimated 85 percent of the cost of IVF.[4] In states requiring insurance coverage for IVF, three times as many couples undergo IVF, but fewer embryos are transferred per cycle, resulting in fewer multiple births.[5] Experts speculate that in states not requiring coverage, there are more multiple births because doctors are under more pressure for "successful" outcomes when people are paying for the procedures out of their own pockets.[6]

Cancer risk. Some couples hesitate to use injectable fertility drugs out of concern that the drugs might cause cancer. In the past, some evidence has suggested a link between fertility drugs and ovarian cancer. But more recent broader studies found no such connection. Another small study demonstrated that women who used human menopausal gonadotropin (HMG, marketed as Pergonal) for six or more months or cycles had an increased risk of breast cancer. This study was not specifically targeted at infertility medications, nor were patients' reports verified through their medical records.[7] Additional larger studies are needed before the actual risk is known. Some groups of infertile women, especially those with endometriosis and unexplained infertility, appear to have a higher-than-normal risk of ovarian cancer, but that increased risk may have to do with the underlying causes that necessitated the medications rather than the medications themselves.[8]

IVF and Its Related Procedures

If using injectables with intercourse or IUI fails to result in a viable pregnancy, or if tubal disease is present, the physician may recommend trying ARTs. While approximately 13 percent of American women will receive infertility services during their lifetime,[9] only 1 to 2 percent of the total female population will undergo treatment with ARTs, which account for about 1 percent of total U.S. births. Despite that small percentage, since 1985, about one million children have been born worldwide using assisted reproductive technologies.[10]

The total number of ART clinics in the United States rose from 30 in 1985 to 421 in 2001.[11] And the number of infants born as a result of ART procedures rose from 1,875 in 1987 (the first year for which statistics were collected) to 40,687 in 2001. The proportion of procedures resulting in pregnancy has also risen from 11.5 percent in 1985 to 32.8 percent in 2001.[12] Not all couples who are candidates feel IVF and its variations are right for them. But for others, it provides a last chance to "be fruitful and multiply."

Just how successful are IVF and its related procedures? The Centers for Disease Control (CDC) and the American Society for Reproductive Medicine (ASRM) publish national IVF success rates two years after the fact. This delay is because pregnancy takes nine months from conception to "measurable outcome." And it takes time after that to collect and process the data. In general, success rates have been on the rise since the inception of IVF, and they average about 25 percent per cycle in the United States across all procedures and age groups. Patients considering IVF should study the latest clinic-specific reports to find the best programs for their particular ages and scenarios.[13]

Of the 107,587 ART cycles reported for 2001, 32.8 percent of those in which fresh nondonor eggs or embryos were used resulted in clinical pregnancies and 40,687 infants born.[14] Twelve percent were multiple-fetus pregnancies.

The risk of multiple births is of considerable concern to couples facing IVF. In addition to the physical risks, multiple births have resulted in "significant decreases in maternal quality of life, health and functioning, and marital satisfaction. Some mothers actually regretted ever seeking IVF treatment after having to cope with more than one baby."[15] This is an important reason to limit the number of eggs fertilized in an ART cycle. Also, compared with naturally conceived singletons, single IVF babies are twice as likely to be born before thirty-seven weeks' gestation and three times more likely to be born before thirty-two weeks. Single IVF babies were three times more likely to have very low birthweights and were slightly more likely to encounter other birth complications. Still, the risk of an IVF singleton being born before thirty-two weeks is small—one or two in 100 births.[16]

> We weren't comfortable trying ARTs, and IVF was the only other option recommended. We both came to the conclusion that it was time to stop. That was the most difficult decision I have ever made. It felt like I was ripping my body apart with my own hands.

> We tried IVF and found to our shock that my husband's healthy-looking sperm wouldn't penetrate my eggs. We could have tried several other options at that point, but none of them appealed to us. Still, we didn't feel we'd wasted the money. We finally had an answer to why this was not happening for us.

> On my first attempt at conception using ARTs I got pregnant. And with only one embryo! They retrieved fifteen eggs, only four were mature, two fertilized, and only one grew. But today that one embryo is four months old and starting to roll over.

The Process of IVF

In vitro fertilization is the foundational ART procedure. The protocol is relatively straightforward, involving three stages: ovulation (either induction with medication or monitoring the process of natural ovulation), retrieval (or harvest), and transfer. Patients should know that there is some variation within the IVF process, as doctors may prescribe no medications or a variety of medications, and they'll exercise some flexibility in the day-to-day recommendations.[17]

Ovulation Induction

In a typical case, before beginning ovarian stimulation, we actually "turn off" the ovaries by using an approach that diminishes messenger hormones from the pituitary. Protocols may include birth control pills, gonadotropin-releasing hormone (GnRH), or both. Ultrasound examination of the ovaries is used to verify that no follicles are maturing, meaning the woman's body is ready for ovarian stimulation. Next, the lab tests her blood for estradiol (one type of estrogen), which will be monitored to determine when the estradiol level is satisfactory.

The patient then starts getting one of the injectables. The medical team determines the type and the daily dosage. Between one and three ampules of the hormone are injected daily for several days, and then the blood's estrogen level is checked again. This level and the size and number of follicles will be monitored as the woman's eggs mature and prepare for ovulation. Most patients take injectables for about ten days.

When the follicles reach sufficient size, the patient then receives an HCG shot to mimic the natural surge in LH. This shot usually triggers ovulation in about thirty-six hours.

Egg Retrieval

About thirty-four hours after the HCG injection, the egg retrieval, or egg harvest, is done using ultrasound and needle aspiration.[18] The ultrasound probe inserted into the vagina for this procedure is equipped with a needle guide. This permits the operator both to see the pelvic structures and to slide the needle into the tiny follicle cysts while observing the process on the screen. By injecting a tiny amount of fluid through the needle into the follicle and then suctioning the fluid, the operator can "wash" or "flush" the mature egg out of the follicle with remarkable proficiency.

Once the operator has aspirated each follicle, the collected fluid is passed to the laboratory. The fluid collected from each follicle is examined for the presence of an egg. Every egg is placed into its own separate sterile container with appropriate supporting medium and is incubated in a sterile environment. The husband's semen sample is collected, evaluated, and processed.

One protocol calls for exposing the eggs to healthy sperm four to six hours after egg retrieval. In cases where the sperm count is low or the number of normally formed sperm is limited, additional procedures (such as intracytoplasmic sperm injection, or ICSI) can be arranged.

The day after the eggs are exposed to sperm, they are evaluated for signs of fertilization. Roughly two out of three eggs will fertilize. We call these fertilized eggs or embryos "zygotes"—human beings at the one-cell stage. While there is ongoing debate about the "personhood" of zygotes,[19] all parties agree that every human began as a zygote and differentiated from that point. No additional genetic material is added after this stage. The only change is in maturation, growth, cell division, and differentiation of different body tissues and supportive structures.

An embryologist identifies and rates, or "grades," the embryos from A to D or 1 to 4 based on appearance and evidence of trauma to the surrounding, supporting structures. Grade A (or 1) embryos are perfect; grade D (or 4) embryos have retarded development. B and C (or 2 and 3) embryos fall in the middle.

By the second day after IVF, the viable embryos have undergone cell division.[20] They are now two- to four-celled beings. The embryologist can observe them under the microscope and identify the growing, healthy embryos. Not all zygotes survive.

Embryo Transfer

By day two, the patient can return for embryo transfer. This process is fairly quick and painless. To block the body's normal cramping response, however, the patient may take ibuprofen or even receive mild sedation. She also receives her first progesterone injection. Progesterone is the body's hormone that "settles the uterus" to keep it from contracting and expelling an early pregnancy. It is often given on the day of egg retrieval and continued through the first ten to twelve weeks of pregnancy or until it is confirmed that no pregnancy occurred.

The embryos are transferred to the uterus using a tiny catheter that deposits them precisely in the uterine cavity. Some researchers have found higher pregnancy rates when doctors measure the length and depth of the uterine cavity with transvaginal ultrasound before embryo transfer so they place embryos precisely.[21]

Most patients report minimal discomfort but are required to rest for several hours after the transfer. Many wonder if further bed rest would increase the odds of pregnancy, but a variety of studies have confirmed that after an initial twenty-minute rest period after transfer, further bed rest does not increase chances of pregnancy.[22]

An increasing number of clinics offer blastocyst transfer (BT) to achieve higher pregnancy rates in difficult cases. This means they must wait longer before performing the embryo transfer. The main reason for this approach is that it allows for the selection of the most developmentally competent and morphologically (structurally) normal embryos. The zygote continues to divide over the first few days of life and can be maintained in the lab for several days. By about day five after fertilization, the tiny human has reached the blastocyst stage, which looks like a hollow ball of cells with a secondary cluster of cells on the inner wall at one end. The inner group of cells will develop into the baby, while the outer sphere becomes the supporting structures such as the placenta and the amniotic sac. Currently only 20 to 40 percent of human embryos survive in the lab to the blastocyst stage, but when blastocysts are transferred to the uterus, they have a high success rate.[23]

We did blastocyst transfer, but we found that there is a lot of "gray" surrounding the issues. It is certainly difficult for couples who have minimal knowledge of what is going on to make these decisions. Our doctor was not a Christian, so he was having a difficult time understanding why we were struggling with this. He kept using the phrase "nonviable embryos," and we could not understand if that meant that they were actually not living or if the embryos just did not look good enough for his standards.

It is generally difficult to get good numbers of high-quality blastocysts with current culture conditions, so new culture media are currently being developed. An improvement in cultures could make blastocyst transfer a viable option for all IVF clinics. One option being explored is co-culture. This involves growing embryos on top of a layer of cells (such as those from the patient's fallopian tube or uterine lining) rather than directly on the bottom of a plastic culture dish. These cells from the patient might help stimulate the development of the embryos. At this point co-culture and blastocyst growth techniques are still experimental, but several published studies have demonstrated improved pregnancy rates and delivery rates (including an increase in births of identical twins[24]) with utilization of co-culture for IVF.[25]

The average age of women undergoing IVF is thirty-five, with 12 percent of women being treated over the age of forty. Because pregnancy rates decline and miscarriage rates rise with age, IVF costs per live birth are more than triple those for women aged forty and older compared with women aged thirty or younger.[26] IVF pregnancy rates depend primarily on the age of the eggs. Our intention in giving these statistics is *not* to discourage you if you are forty or older but to inform you as you prayerfully decide what procedures best fit your ethics and how to best use your available resources.

Studies using younger egg donors for older women demonstrate the enormous significance of the egg's age.[27] As a result, some clinics offer donor eggs, which improve the take-home baby rates for older candidates. Women who conceive using donor eggs must keep in mind that the offspring share no genetic connection with the biological (or birth) mother. We'll explore the ethics of third-party reproduction in the next few chapters.

When considering a specific clinic's success rates, factor in whether or not that facility treats patients over forty and the average number of embryos that are transferred in a cycle. Clinics that treat women over forty will have lower success rates, even though their expertise may be first-rate. A clinic's higher success rate may simply reflect a focus on treating younger patients and rejecting more difficult cases.

At present, sperm freezing and thawing procedures are effective. Though a significant number of sperm die in the process, sperm are generally so numerous that even with the loss of many, the remaining ones are quite capable of fertilizing eggs. Unfortunately, current technology is far less efficient at freezing and thawing eggs, despite considerable efforts to solve this problem.

In the course of normal human fertilization, conception occurs in the fallopian tube, and the first cell divisions take place while the embryo is still in the tube. It has been suggested that some vital chemical communication that facilitates implantation takes place in the tube as the developing embryo travels to the uterine cavity. The embryo spends several days in the tube and then several more days in the uterus before implanting. Thus, while some researchers focused their attention on exploring the complexities of IVF, others explored the possibility of using the woman's tubes (assuming they're healthy) to assist in the process and came up with different but related procedures. The result was GIFT and ZIFT.

GIFT (gamete intrafallopian transfer). GIFT involves the same process of ovulation induction we described earlier. The physician harvests the eggs by ultrasound-guided aspiration, and a sperm sample is prepared. The gametes (sperm and egg) are then placed into a syringe-catheter apparatus. Using laparoscopic technique, the doctor injects the fluid containing sperm and a designated number of eggs into the fallopian tube. This provides the opportunity for fertilization to occur naturally in the tube. When the procedure works, normal cell division occurs in the tube and the embryo arrives on schedule for implantation in the awaiting uterus. Appropriate hormonal support is used to optimize the environment.

While the GIFT patient may go through hyperstimulation of the ovaries to produce more eggs, the number of eggs injected can be controlled, thereby decreasing the risk of multiple births. Though any zygote can split into identical twins or even triplets, the occurrence of multiple births is minimized with GIFT.[28]

ZIFT (zygote intrafallopian transfer). With GIFT, we don't know for certain that fertilization took place until we have a positive pregnancy test. With ZIFT, the medical team obtains the sperm and egg in the same way, but the eggs are exposed to the sperm outside the body, in the culture dish. Once fertilization occurs and a one-celled human being (zygote) is established, the physician uses laparoscopic surgery to gently inject this zygote into the fallopian tube. Hormonal support is provided, and cell division takes place in the tube and in the uterus before normal implantation.

In skilled hands, both GIFT and ZIFT are effective approaches. The pregnancy rates for these procedures are relatively good, but they do require the presence of normal fallopian tubes.

Which is best? In cases of tubal damage, disease, or congenital absence, GIFT and ZIFT are out of the question. Most fertility centers gain expertise in one approach or the other and specialize in that approach. Each couple needs to assess their particular circumstances and decide on the best approach with the help of their medical team. The trend today is away from GIFT and ZIFT and toward IVF.

Today the infertility business is a $2.7 billion industry. It started in 1978 with the first "test-tube baby," Louise Brown. Since then, the process of allowing the union of sperm and egg to happen in vitro (that is, in glass) has become more common. Brown's father's sperm fertilized her mother's egg in a tissue-culture dish. Within thirty-six hours, scientists transferred the fertilized egg to her mother's womb (in vitro fertilization–embryo transfer, IVF-ET), and the embryo grew. In the decades since then, doctors have come up with many variations of this process.

Micromanipulation

In addition to IVF, GIFT, and ZIFT, we have the following micromanipulation techniques for overcoming infertility.

ICSI (intracytoplasmic sperm injection). Perhaps the most dramatic micromanipulation procedure is ICSI, which can aid husbands with low sperm counts or men whose sperm have difficulty penetrating the egg. More than 20,000 ICSI babies have been born since its development in Belgium in the early 1990s.

With ICSI, the doctor retrieves maturing eggs from the woman and obtains and prepares a sperm sample. The embryologist then selects a single, normal-appearing, vigorously swimming sperm and loads it into a pipette, which serves as a microscopic injecting apparatus. Having stabilized the egg, the embryologist then pierces the thin tissue and injects the sperm into the egg's cytoplasm.

At this point, the genetic material of the sperm must align with the egg's. Somehow the egg knows penetration has occurred, and its genetic material located in the nucleus unravels and aligns with the male chromosomes.

Doctors using this procedure have absolute control over the potential number of embryos created, so it does not present the usual worries about unintended multiple pregnancies, nor must couples face the decision of whether or not to cryopreserve, or freeze, "extra" embryos.

We see some conflicting evidence about the risk to children born via ICSI, which has raised some concerns about this procedure. Whereas during normal conception, only the strongest sperm make the long journey and break through the membrane of the egg to fertilize it, ICSI bypasses this natural process, and the weakest and strongest sperm are never separated.

A 2002 study found that infertile men who have normal-looking sperm may actually have unseen DNA damage. It is believed that this damage interferes both with attempts to conceive a child and with a child's future health. Researchers concluded that infertility specialists need to look more closely at the sperm of men who have trouble conceiving. Though about one-quarter of the infertile men studied had normal-looking sperm, a high percentage of these sperm had DNA damage. If such a damaged sperm is used to fertilize an egg, the result may be anything from a failure to conceive or a miscarriage to a child with abnormalities. The test group was relatively small, but the findings suggest a need for further research.[29] Clearly, the selection of the sperm is an enormous responsibility.

Additionally, the placement of the sperm within the egg can be risky. But a developing technology—an instrument that illuminates the inner structure of an egg—may allow fertility specialists to improve outcomes. Because scientists can't see the chromosomes inside an egg, sperm cells are sometimes injected in a way that damages the egg's DNA. Doctors are finding, however, that a polarized light device can reveal the location of the genetic material inside the egg without harming the egg itself.[30]

ROSNI (round spermatic nuclear injection) and MESA (microscopic epididymal sperm aspiration. A man can have a zero sperm count but still make sperm. That's because the "plumbing"—the tubes that bring the sperm from the testicle—can fail to develop properly. In fact, a key part of the tubing called the vas deferens can fail to develop at all, leaving sperm forever in the testicle to die and dissolve. Today doctors can harvest these immature sperm by needle aspiration, either of the testes (ROSNI)[31] or of the existing ductwork (MESA). The resulting sperm can be used with ICSI to achieve fertilization.

Assisted hatching. Another option is called "assisted hatching." The human egg has a shell—not a thick calcium structure like the shell of a chicken egg, but a thicker, tougher layer of surrounding cells. As a woman ages, her released eggs have tougher shells. Back in the early 1990s, a theory emerged that some patients failed to have successful outcomes following IVF because the embryo couldn't escape (hatch) from its shell. So doctors began to assist in this "hatching" process by mechanically or chemically making a small hole in the shell right before embryo transfer.

Candidates for this technique are women who are over thirty-eight, have high FSH levels, have had previous failed in vitro cycles, are doing ICSI, and/or are using frozen and thawed embryos. There is some evidence that in these selected cases, assisted hatching increases the number of embryos that implant.

When I looked into the available ARTs, I felt overwhelmed with what seemed like alphabet soup—IVF, GIFT, ZIFT, ROSNI, ICSI.

It's hard to read clinic success rates. If a program specializes in hard cases, the rates may look less impressive, while they're actually practicing cutting-edge medicine. That's why it's important to network with consumer groups such as RESOLVE and INCIID. They can help interpret the figures.

Infertility Fraud

In addition to the procedural and ethical questions couples have about ARTs, there are other concerns, as well. How ethical and "safe" are the clinics? We've all heard about infertility clinic horror stories. Here's a sampling:

- An embryologist was found guilty of eight counts of falsifying records at two clinics and, following an audit, was also found to still be storing thirty-nine embryos that he had pretended to transfer.
- A doctor offered free IVF treatment to women who were desperate to have a baby on the condition that they donate some of their eggs to his clinic.
- A woman gave birth to two infants—one black and one white—after she was impregnated with the embryo of another couple along with her own embryos. The black child's parents won custody of the black child. The woman lost an appeal in which she sought visitation rights.
- A couple gave birth to twins after the woman was impregnated with what she thought were embryos from her eggs and her husband's sperm. Both infants were later discovered to have B-positive blood types—a genetic impossibility for parents who both have O-positive blood types. The woman's eggs had been fertilized with the wrong sperm.

Though such reports get our attention, they're relatively rare. It has been estimated that the likelihood of such a mix-up is about one in six hundred (based on one in six cycles producing a baby, and assuming one error in every one hundred cycles). We bring them up only to remind couples of the need to be fully informed of the risks when considering high-tech procedures.

There are other risks, as well. Stories abound about divorced couples who sue to have embryos destroyed or thawed and transferred against the wishes of former partners. There are also the risks we already mentioned—for example, the risk of birth defects for children conceived through ICSI. But what about the broader group of babies born via IVF? Emerging studies from reputable institutions have found preliminary evidence of birth defects and genetic abnormalities. Larger studies are needed to conclusively determine whether an increased risk does exist, and in fact, additional research is underway. Experts are looking at a number of reports that express concern that ICSI, egg freezing, and embryo freezing may be linked to higher rates of birth defects than with natural conception. To date, any increased incidence of additional risk has been shown to be very small.

While some groups have been quick to use these studies as conclusive proof that couples should avoid IVF, many at the opposite end of the spectrum have discounted the studies. Perhaps the truth lies somewhere between the two poles. Preliminary studies are just that—preliminary.

There is, however, one piece of clearly good news. Research suggests that IVF babies' families are stable and strong. In fact, couples who have had a child with some high-tech help have marriages that are as strong or stronger than couples who have not struggled with infertility. And children conceived through ARTs appear to have normal behavioral development. A research team from Australia compared five-year-old children conceived through IVF and ICSI with children conceived naturally and found no differences in child behavior or development between the two groups.[32]

For thousands of couples who have attempted IVF using their own eggs and sperm, the result has been a take-home baby. Their photos line the walls of IVF clinics.

DISCUSSION QUESTIONS

1. Do you think you and your spouse are good candidates for IVF? Why or why not?
2. Does the clinic you're considering belong to SART (Society for Assisted Reproductive Technology)?
3. How long has the clinic been doing ARTs?
4. What are its success rates for people in your age and treatment category?
5. How many transfers per month are performed at the clinic?
6. Do the doctors respect your personal convictions about the status of the human embryo?
7. What percentage of the clinic's patients have multiple births? How do you feel about multiple births?
8. Does the clinic have a waiting list? If so, how long is it?
9. What will it cost you to do a complete IVF cycle? What will it cost if you have to cancel after a partial cycle?
10. Is counseling available?
11. Can you talk with other patients who have been through the clinic's program?
12. How would you pay for an IVF cycle? Do you have insurance coverage? Family support?

Chapter 13

A Moral Minefield

We Can Do It, but Should We?

I had a whole string of early pregnancy losses. The doctor recommended chromosome and antibody analyses, but they turned up nothing. We began investigating assisted reproductive technologies (ARTs). Although the success rates seemed low, even if we didn't achieve a pregnancy, we wondered what we might learn from the process. Maybe our embryos were staying inside the tube and not making it into the uterus. Can a Christian use such medical treatments, or is that "taking matters into our own hands"?

We didn't put a lot of thought into the "right and wrong" of what we were doing. We wanted a baby. We wanted to give the gift of a child to each other, and either of us probably would have sacrificed anything if we thought it would result in a success.

How many to fertilize, what to do with "leftover embryos," whether we'd consider using a donor, destroying embryos without thinking— answering those questions beforehand saved my husband and me a lot of stress while in the midst of in vitro fertilization (IVF).

The deep desire for children is part of the divine design. Yet the Bible doesn't address ARTs. So are we left on our own with no biblical guidance? Couples in treatment face tough moral choices that have the potential to add enormous guilt to the pain of infertility. How far can or should a couple go technologically to have a child? What are the moral issues? When we explore these questions, we enter the realm of bioethics—the morality of health care. It concerns the "right and wrong" of certain medical options. While medicine often raises the question, "Can we do it?" ethics and morality ask, "Should we?"

Right or Wrong—Who Decides?

In our postmodern age, many people deny the existence of absolute truth. That is, they believe there's never an absolute right or wrong—what one person sees as ethical, another might see as immoral—and both can be right at the same time, since nothing is absolute. (Ironically, "nothing is absolute" is itself an absolute statement.) Christians take Scripture, inspired by the Creator God, as absolute. Practices that the Scriptures declare to be wrong, such as murder, then, are clearly wrong.

Most of us feel competent to discern right from wrong, good from bad. Yet we quickly discover that in simpler spheres such as music, movies, and even appearance, it's impossible to achieve a consensus. If we asked people to name good and bad movies from the previous year, we'd get a variety of answers—some of them argued forcefully.

When we consider medical options, good people—even those who hold to biblical absolutes—often disagree. How far is too far? How can those who believe in Christ and his Word come to different conclusions? Might God guide a couple in one direction and guide another couple to take an entirely different path? How do we reconcile opposing pronouncements coming from Spirit-led people?

How can we find answers to these complex and significant issues? Scripture reveals some clear nonnegotiables, such as the sanctity of human life and "Do to others as you would have them do to you" (Luke 6:31). But what about the areas where we find no absolutes? We find an example of such a situation in Romans 14, where we learn that first-century Christians disagreed about whether they could eat meat. Some believers considered it wrong to eat meat, perhaps because so much meat in that culture was offered to false gods; others considered it right to demonstrate their faith by eating meat. The apostle Paul referred to the latter as the stronger Christians but concluded that each should live as his or her conscience dictated. Church members were not to judge each other, but rather to show deference to others with whom they disagreed.

People of faith are going to disagree. And they will do so—sometimes emphatically—on practices that relate to infertility treatment. Some churches have clear teachings on issues relating to reproduction; others allow for individual discernment. We encourage each reader to understand the instruction of his or her particular church as part of the decision-making process. When interacting with people of traditions that differ from our own, it's important to avoid making dogmatic statements such as, "No good Christian could ever (fill in the blank with . . .) "do IVF," "freeze embryos," "hire a surrogate."

I had my consultation with my doctor about pursuing IVF. Even Christians have different views on certain issues! Because of problems with my uterus, he wants to fertilize as many eggs as we can—put three in and freeze the rest. I told him my concerns about freezing. He said the ones that make it through the thawing process are the ones that would most likely survive naturally anyway. He said it is rare that we would have any to freeze at all. Because of the cycle day I am on, he wanted to start immediately, but I am still uncomfortable with this. My husband wants to do it the way the doctor recommends. But why won't the doctors respect what I am saying? I think, "Let's just set our boundaries. At least I won't have the moral regret."

In the absence of clear scriptural commands regarding a particular issue, we look for underlying principles. The Old Testament prophet Micah summarized for God's people what the Lord requires: "To do justly, to love mercy, and to walk humbly with your God" (Mic. 6:8 NKJV). Jesus summarized Jewish law by saying it all boils down to "Love the Lord your God with all your heart and with all your soul and with all your mind" and "Love your neighbor as yourself" (Matt. 22:37–39). These commands lay the foundation for our decision making; we ask whether our decisions demonstrate love for God and for others.

How do we find out what demonstrates such love? We discover both the absolutes and the principles for decision making in the Bible. Psalm 19 speaks of how God's Word is perfect, making the simple wise and restoring the soul. In the New Testament, we read that "all Scripture is God-breathed and is useful for teaching, rebuking, correcting and training in righteousness," so that godly people are equipped for good works (2 Tim. 3:16–17). The word "useful" could also be translated "beneficial." This suggests a degree of flexibility in addressing varying eras and cultures. Thus, the Scriptures provide the stories, principles, and precepts we need to help us live God-honoring lives. Christians have the additional benefit of God's indwelling Spirit to guide them (John 16:13).

Most people in treatment desire to do what's right, but they lack guidance in knowing what it means to do right during infertility treatment. Thus, in this chapter, we will consider scriptural principles and how they relate to decision making in infertility treatment. Then in the next chapter, we will move on to the field of ethics to help provide a framework for decision-making when in treatment.

At the beginning of our struggle I honestly didn't think about ethics. But we had to sign papers before a retrieval and transfer. One paper asked us what to do with the embryos that weren't going to make it.

The first IVF, we said discard. Later I felt horrible knowing that we had discarded life before the embryos were actually done developing. I felt so guilty. But I've repented of my sin, and I believe that God has forgiven me of my ignorance. Our second and third try, we froze all leftover embryos, and we transferred all that survived the thaw.

We wrestled with our IVF decisions, especially the number of eggs to fertilize, and whether or not to freeze. We came to a breaking point at which we said we could no longer make this kind of life-and-death decision. We felt like we were gambling with embryos. So we discontinued treatment after our second IVF.

When we bring up the ethics of infertility treatment, people often ask, "Isn't using ARTs playing God?" As a noted theologian has pointed out, unless scientists start commanding matter to emerge from nothingness, we're in no danger of anyone "playing God" anytime soon, at least in the creative sense. Yet it *is* possible to overstep the boundaries he has set and thus enter a realm rightfully reserved only for him.

So we begin by asking, What boundaries *has* God set?

Respect the Sanctity of Human Life

A fundamental question we must consider when we explore the ethics of ARTs is, When does human life begin? Life begins when egg and sperm unite, followed within twenty-four hours by the alignment and activation of their DNA. At this point, the embryo begins to function as an integrated whole. The unique person, with all its genetic complement, is present from the moment of DNA alignment and activation. Assuming a later time of ensoulment based on a purely arbitrary timeline and thus allowing for the destruction of zygotes probably oversteps the boundaries of the dominion that God has given to humans.[1]

Theologically, most evangelicals believe that both the material (physical) and immaterial (spiritual) elements of humanity are transmitted through sexual reproduction, rather than believing that these elements are transmitted in two distinct moments—physical creation and a later ensoulment. Thus, it is believed that children inherit immaterial as well as material traits from their parents.[2] While God did breathe life into the first human after he was formed from the dust, there is no parallel ensoulment event in the woman's creation.

So how are we to treat human life? We read in Genesis 1 about the first man and woman, whom he pronounced "very good," the crown jewels of his creation: "God blessed them and said to them, 'Be fruitful and increase in number; fill the earth and subdue it. Rule over the fish of the sea and the birds of the air and over every living creature that moves on the ground'" (Gen. 1:28).

The Hebrew word for "living creature" refers to animal life and is often used for four-legged beasts. So when God outlined the boundaries of human dominion, he gave the man and woman dominion over the plant, fish, and animal kingdoms. Notice that something's missing from this list: other human beings. While we might kill fish to eat, we abhor cannibalism; we might experiment on mice, but we believe we shouldn't destroy human life to benefit humanity. Humans are special. And killing humans is contrary to God's revelation.

From the first human cell stage (zygote) to the approximately thirty trillion cells in the full-grown person, every cell gets its genetic code from that first cell. Thus, every human being develops by beginning as a zygote following a "living DNA blueprint" that does not fundamentally change with maturity. We have a continuity of this genetic material throughout life. The one-celled life represents the human being in its tiniest, most vulnerable form and requires our respectful treatment.

What about Fertility Drugs?

We see from a variety of Scripture passages that we may seek to overcome some effects of the Fall by working to cure diseases. Thus, in the same way we would support using antibiotics for infections and chemotherapy for cancers, we feel it is appropriate to advise couples to use medical intervention to treat fertility problems.

At a time when anesthetics, painkillers, and mood elevators were unavailable, strong drink was recommended for the suffering (Prov. 31:6–7). The Good Samaritan parable, recorded by Luke, shows that we are to try to help the injured (Luke 10:25–37). Jesus sent the disciples to heal the sick (Matt. 10:8). Paul told Timothy to take something to treat his stomach problems (1 Tim. 5:23). While it's true that the woman with the "issue of blood" had suffered much at the hands of physicians (Mark 5:26), Jesus said that those who are well don't need a physician, *but the sick do* (Matt. 9:12, italics ours). In fact, in his earthly ministry, Jesus used touch, spittle, and the recommendation to bathe in connection with supernatural healing. In short, a biblical worldview allows for the practice of good medicine as long as one doesn't trust *only* in doctors as King Asa did (2 Chron. 16:12).

Depending on a patient's underlying medical condition, we could label many medications as fertility drugs. For example, for a man with a prostate infection, a simple course of antibiotics could be considered fertility treatment. For a woman with low thyroid, replacement hormone would represent a fertility drug. Based on the premise that drug therapy qualifies as a moral practice, taking many of such medicines (e.g., antibiotics, thyroid medication) would qualify as fertility treatment.

Part of assessing the right and wrong of prescription drugs, however, is factoring in the degree of acceptable risk. In medicine, it's called the risk-benefit ratio, and it is considered when recommending any kind of intervention.[3]

Three weeks after my doctor put me on Lupron, I was in the emergency room with migraines so bad that they thought I was having strokes. My MRI did, in fact, show that I had a small stroke. I discontinued Lupron and have lived with neurosurgeries every six to nine months from that point until this very day.

Even if a medication is legal, we must determine if the risk of taking it is appropriate for us.

Some have argued that because infertility is a matter of "God closing the womb" (as was true of Sarah, Hannah, Elizabeth), faith alone must be sufficient in overcoming infertility. Others believe that, while he is able to open and close wombs, God has permitted us only limited insight into the complex functioning of the human body. Recognizing that approximately 90 percent of infertility cases stem from diagnosable medical conditions and that approximately 60 percent of couples pursuing treatment will go on to experience live birth, many argue that medical therapy for infertility is appropriate as long as no one violates scriptural principles.

All of this suggests that we can trust God *and* use medicine, as long as we value all life in the process. Humans are made of both spirit and matter, with both being equally real. Thus, a Christian patient may take medicine to overcome a thyroid problem; a Christian woman may use ovulation inducers for underactive ovaries; a Christian couple may explore the variety of medical options available to them. Yet medicine has its moral limits. If, in the hope of finding cures for disease, we go so far as to snuff out life (donating embryos to stem-cell research, for example), we move beyond the areas in which we've been given dominion and enter a realm reserved for the Divine.

We struggled with ethical decisions. We didn't want to make choices we'd later regret. We prayed, asked opinions, researched, weighed the odds, and talked with our doctor. We had to hold life in any form in highest regard; if life was created, we were totally responsible for it, period. The first decision was whether even to do IVF. Next we examined, "When does life begin?" The moment of conception? When the genetic material actually is mixed? When it first divides? When it becomes a six-cell embryo? Implantation? All evidence points to fertilization. Next we decided, To freeze or not to freeze? If we didn't want to freeze and our doctor would transfer only three or four embryos, we would have to make sure only three or four viable embryos were created.

What about "Artificial" Procedures?

Most couples have few questions about the morality of taking medication or going through an infertility workup. Only when they face IVF and its related procedures do they begin to ask many more questions. That is probably because, as bioethics expert Dr. Leon Kass has noted, "At stake is the idea of the humanness of our human life and the meaning of our embodiment, our sexual being, and our relation to ancestors and descendants."[4]

For the Christian proceeding with IVF, holding a high view of human life (even at the embryo stage) and respecting the boundaries of our dominion will impact what is approved in the IVF lab and afterward. Life and death matters are at stake when we move to considering the ethics of ARTs. Such questions as determining when human life begins become more than academic discussions. They're critical points in deciding what to do with "excess" embryos, embryos that are graded as being of poor quality, frozen embryos, and even experimentation on embryos and so-called pre-embryos.

At this point, we will define some key terms that will help patients seeking to honor the sanctity of human life.

Is a pre-embryo a human life? Yes, a so-called pre-embryo is a human life, not a prelife form, or tissue in a prefertilization form. Because the term "pre-embryo" is confusing, we prefer to avoid it, but patients do need to know what it means. A pre-embryo is the product of the union of egg-and-sperm (embryo) from the time of fertilization until it is fourteen days old. This overlaps with the term "embryo," which refers to the tiny human life from the time of fertilization through the age of eight weeks.

Pre-embryo: first two weeks of life

Embryo: first eight weeks of life

The term "pre-embryo" was introduced in 1986, primarily for reasons of public policy. It often conveys the erroneous idea that a new human is formed at some time *well after* fertilization, to fit the concept that humanity, and thus personhood, begins not at fertilization but at implantation or some time after that. This gives physicians and scientists at IVF clinics some leeway in how they can treat these tiny, developing humans. It keeps them from having to publicize the deaths of two-cell, four-cell, and eight-cell humans, which are common occurrences in IVF labs.[5]

Back in the early 1990s, a woman who was highly involved in influencing public policy rhetoric enthusiastically described how she had convinced a pro-lifer to support research on human embryos. She had done so, she said, by using the word "pre-embryo," convincing him that he should not oppose research on the pre-embryo because it was not yet alive.

Do conception, implantation, and fertilization differ? Yes. Since 1972, the American Medical Association has officially defined "conception" as being synonymous with "implantation," which is clearly different from "fertilization."

Fertilization occurs when the sperm penetrates the egg. About a week later, the embryo's growing collection of cells nestles into the wall of the uterus (womb), an event technically called "implantation" and now also referred to as "conception." Many pro-lifers who say "Human life begins at conception" are unaware of this subtle difference and actually mean to say "Life begins at fertilization," which happens about a week prior to conception/implantation. So it's important to define these terms.[6]

"Conception" and "fertilization" are not synonyms, according to current medical dictionaries. In addition, doctors do not "implant" embryos into the uterus following IVF; they transfer them, though often even medical writers in the media use "implant" when they mean "transfer."

Decisions about the ethics of many available technological advancements hinge on understanding and communicating precisely with the unique vocabulary of each specialty. So we will proceed in the next chapter by defining some terms and principles related to bioethics, and then we'll explore the ethical questions associated with high-tech treatment.

DISCUSSION QUESTIONS

1. Discuss your views about the value of human life, even at the earliest stage.
2. Many clinics strongly suggest that all IVF patients maximize egg harvest by creating multiple embryos. How do you feel about this creation of "extra" embryos?
3. About half of all frozen embryos die during the thawing process. Is this number acceptable to you?
4. What will you do with "extra" embryos if your family size is complete but embryos remain?
5. How do you feel about third-party arrangements: donor egg, donor sperm, surrogacy, and embryo adoption?
6. Why do you feel that way? Does your spouse agree? Your family? Your faith family?

Chapter 14

DETERMINING RIGHT FROM WRONG

THE ETHICS CONSTRUCT

Couples making decisions about reproductive technologies come from a variety of church traditions with differing teachings on these matters. We encourage each person to obey his or her conscience and to stay within the boundaries of his or her denomination. Yet because there is often a great deal of liberty allowed within various traditions, we offer for consideration four principles that are used in a secular approach to ethical decision making.

We will begin by establishing a common vocabulary, using basic accepted terminology in the field of ethics. In the widely used text *Principles of Biomedical Ethics*, the authors highlight four major ethical principles that help to facilitate discussion about complex bioethical concerns.[1] Developed in a nonreligious framework, these four principles provide a vocabulary for many of the debates about new technology. The Christian can use them with ease because they are consistent with a biblical worldview. The four principles (to which we will refer collectively as the "construct") are as follows:

- *Beneficence*—to do good. Thus, we ask, "Does it do good?"
- *Nonmaleficence*—to do no harm. We ask, "Does it avoid doing harm?"
- *Autonomy*—the patient has the right to make decisions about care rendered to him or her. We ask, "Does it respect self-determination, the patient's right to decide for him- or herself?"[2]
- *Justice*—fair, equitable, and appropriate distribution of social benefits and burdens. Our own definition of justice goes beyond this definition to ask whether something seeks what is right or due the patient in a given instance. So we ask, "Does it give what is right, due, and equitable?"

When making decisions about treatment, couples should consider their options in light of this construct. To demonstrate, let's consider whether it would be acceptable to use thyroid medication for overcoming an imbalance. First, we ask if the goal in taking the medicine is to do good. Yes, restoring normal functioning to the body is a good goal. Second, does taking such medicine avoid harm? Yes, it contributes to the overall health of the individual. Third, does it respect the right of the patient to decide for him- or herself? Certainly, if the patient makes the decision about taking the medication (rather than having someone sneak it into her soup). Finally, is it just? Perhaps one does not have a *right* to take the medication, but certainly taking it would not be an *un*just act. According to the construct, taking thyroid medication is ethical.

By asking the four questions outlined above, a patient can often determine what is appropriate. Yet occasionally when a decision involves more than one life, we may face a conflict of interest. For example, what if to do good to one does harm to another? Is abortion okay when the mother will die without it? Does one weigh and prioritize such questions based on a "lesser" or "greater" evil or good? Or does the answer depend on the situation? We prefer more precision than that! We want black and white, right and wrong.

Following are the most common questions related to infertility diagnosis and treatment, followed by an assessment using the four-question construct.

Is it okay to produce a semen sample? A consideration for Roman Catholics here is whether it's okay to separate ejaculation from procreation (see chapter 8). If the two are inseparably linked, producing a semen sample by masturbation is unacceptable. Yet those who see sexual intimacy as having no unitive-procreative requirement proceed by considering the decision in light of the ethics construct we have set out:

- *Good?* Producing a semen sample is done with a good goal in mind—that of having a child. Producing a sample will possibly help with the diagnosis.
- *Harm?* It does no harm unless the husband violates the lust parameters mentioned in chapter 9.
- *Autonomy?* A man is deciding of his own free will to produce a sample.
- *Justice?* Producing a sample is legal and does not violate anyone's rights.

Based on these ethical parameters, we conclude it is acceptable to produce a sample.

Some doctors grow frustrated when patients' decisions of conscience might negatively impact their clinic success rates. As a result, some doctors have insisted that treating the embryo as life is as illogical as treating the sperm or egg as life. But sperm has only half the necessary DNA to make up a human being. It is alive, but it is not a life.

Is it okay to use fertility drugs?

- *Good?* Conception is a good goal.
- *Harm?* Known risks are hyperstimulation of the ovaries, excessive ovarian growth, and effects on blood clotting. There is also a small bit of evidence that links fertility drugs with cancer. The husband and wife weigh these risks against the benefits and determine whether they can accept the risks. Roman Catholics, Protestants, and Jewish people alike usually approve of fertility medications because the drugs are designed to improve the normal ovarian process of producing an egg.
- *Autonomy?* Patients must be free to make the decision after being fully informed of both the benefits and the risks.
- *Justice?* The medications prescribed are legal and permissible. Cost issues may impact some decisions. Neither insurance companies nor the state are required to pay for medications.

Is surgery okay? As with medications, "fertility surgery" may be broadly defined. Doing an appendectomy on a female patient before the appendix ruptures classifies as a fertility operation, because if her appendix ruptures, the patient's odds of infertility problems dramatically increase. Surgery to restore normal anatomy to a damaged tube or a vas deferens that has not formed properly would be acceptable according to the ethical construct.

Let's consider a specific surgical procedure—microsurgical epididymal sperm aspiration (MESA)—in which immature sperm are harvested from the epididymis:

- *Good?* Having a child is a good goal.
- *Harm?* A patient must consider the potential for failure (success rates vary significantly depending on the wife's age) and infection. As of this writing, there is no known risk to children who would be born.
- *Autonomy?* The patient understands the risks and benefits.
- *Justice?* It's legal. Is MESA *due* the patient? Neither insurance companies nor the state has any obligation to make it available. While MESA may be unavailable in many parts of the world, no ethical reason prohibits patients from proceeding.

Caution

Is artificial insemination using my husband's sperm okay? Some people who vehemently oppose artificial insemination have confused it with in vitro fertilization or donor insemination. With artificial insemination, the doctor deposits sperm in the vagina near the cervix or directly into the uterus (IUI—intrauterine insemination) with the use of a syringe. Some Roman Catholic couples actually face less of a moral dilemma over providing semen for IUI than they do when providing it for a routine semenalysis. (To their thinking, at least with IUI, the semen will make it into the uterus.) According to the Vatican, IUI within marriage is unacceptable "except for those cases in which the technical means is not a substitute for the conjugal act but serves to facilitate and to help so that the act attains its natural purpose."[3]

For those who see an inseparable link between the unitive and procreative elements of sex, special condoms would have to be used for collection. For those who see no such link, we offer the following:

- *Good?* Having a child is a good goal.
- *Harm?* There is minimal risk. The most common complications are allergic reaction and infection, which occur only rarely.
- *Autonomy?* An informed patient chooses whether or not to have the procedure done.
- *Justice?* Artificial insemination with husband's sperm is both legal and permissible.

Caution

Is in vitro fertilization (IVF) ethically okay if we respect life at the one-cell stage? If so, what boundaries do we set for our doctor? Couples can do IVF while complying with all ethical principles if they honor life at the one-cell stage. That means deciding that every embryo must get the best possible chance to live.

How can couples make sure every embryo gets such a chance? *They begin by allowing to be created only the number of embryos that they are willing to carry to term in that cycle in the event that all embryos implant.* (Each egg gets its own petri dish, so it's easy to limit the number of eggs exposed to sperm.) When and if fertilization takes place and cell division indicates that DNA has aligned, all embryos—regardless of "quality"—are then transferred, each having an equal chance at being carried to term.[4]

In the hours or days that the embryos are observed before transfer, many do not survive the normal process of cell division. We assume this would have happened in the fallopian tubes under normal circumstances, and the potential parents would never have known the sperm had reached the egg.[5] Embryologists can watch embryos that have questionable growth rates so that only live, or viable, embryos are transferred—up until the blastocyst stage. Any embryo reaching the blastocyst stage should be transferred or frozen for later transfer (see the ethical argument above).

More and more clinics now limit the number of embryos transferred to the number the mother can safely carry to term, recognizing that any or all of the embryos could twin. Limiting the number transferred appears to raise success rates.[6]

Placing limits on the number of embryos transferred helps a couple avoid facing *multifetal pregnancy reduction*, a procedure in which the uterus has more live embryos than it can support, so one (or more) of the fetuses is aborted to make room for the others. (This differs from *selective reduction*, a procedure in which an implanted embryo in a group of two or more other implanted embryos is selected for abortion because it is shown to have abnormalities.) *Both of these procedures involve the destruction of human life and fail the ethical test.*

The best decision is to avoid, as much as possible, situations in which these options would be considered. In other words, limit the number of embryos created and thus limit the number of embryos transferred.

Legislation passed in Sweden in 2003 makes the transfer of a single embryo the overriding rule, with only one in ten transfers allowing transfer of two embryos. In the United States, the transferring of three to five or more embryos is common, though we are seeing a trend toward transferring fewer embryos, which are selected for their higher quality, with more cell divisions.

In summary, as we said, couples can do IVF while complying with all ethical principles, but to do so they must honor life at the one-cell stage.

Caution

Is cryopreservation acceptable? When it comes to determining the morality of freezing, or cryopreserving, embryos, the assessment has two stages. The first is determining the acceptability of freezing embryos that are not to be transferred in an IVF cycle. The second is determining what should be done with frozen embryos that a couple has decided they no longer want to use.

We begin with the first in light of the ethics construct:

- *Good?* Couples choosing cryopreservation to sustain embryos not transferred in an IVF cycle intend to do good—to increase their chances of having children. Freezing embryos can save money and avoid the inconvenience of having to do another IVF cycle. This assumes the couple is committed to subsequently allowing each embryo the opportunity to develop normally within the womb.

- *Harm?* Half of all cryopreserved embryos die in the thawing process. While some say those embryos would have died even without cryopreservation, we have no data to support this claim. We do know that the freeze-thaw process is hard on sperm, because so many of them die. The same is true for eggs. Thus, evidence suggests that the freeze-thaw process is hard on embryos too. Once they survive the thawing process, however, embryos appear to have no long-term effects from cryopreservation.
- *Autonomy?* For the husband and wife, informed consent applies. But now we have a new life at a one-cell stage—a human that has no ability to make a decision as far as accepting the risk. What about the embryo's autonomy? If the embryo could decide, would it choose to be transferred or frozen?
- *Justice?* Justice is served for the potential parents. It would be difficult to make a case that justice is served for the frozen embryo.

If a couple is suddenly faced with seven embryos in the IVF lab, deciding to cryopreserve them is certainly more ethical than discarding "excess" embryos. But it would be better to avoid getting into this situation. Until thaw survival and conception rates improve following cryopreservation, *couples should consider avoiding this situation by allowing sperm to fertilize fewer eggs*, even though the financial cost may be higher as a result.

Depending on what you read, some clinics estimate they have a 50 percent thaw survival rate. Others quote between 60 and 70 percent. Clinics with higher rates may be freezing only the higher quality embryos in the first place (allowing the "lesser" quality embryos to be discarded). These are questions to investigate with the individual clinic, but know that clinics with higher ethical standards may have lower success rates for this reason.

Some researchers have questioned whether the chemicals used and the freezing process in cryopreservation might sometimes alter the embryos' genetics. We don't yet have enough information to know. We do know, however, that several clinics in Great Britain now emphasize doing natural cycle IVF, optimizing the natural cycle rather than using fertility drugs. IVF is much less expensive without the ovulation-induction medications, and while the odds of success in each cycle are lower, couples can try numerous times. Other clinics, especially over- seas, are moving toward limiting transfers to one embryo per IVF cycle.[7]

Ideally, researchers will continue to perfect the process of freezing and thawing eggs. Facing the decision to freeze gametes (eggs and sperm) is less problematic than freezing embryos, because gametes are not live humans, but embryos are. Currently eggs can be frozen, but they are much more fragile than sperm, they don't freeze and thaw well, and there are far fewer of them. The average normal ejaculate has about 60 million sperm per milliliter; the average number of eggs per cycle is one. If you lost 50 million sperm in the freeze-thaw process, you'd still probably have a lot of sperm left; if you lost the same number of frozen eggs, you'd have lost the equivalent of the entire population of Ukraine.

Having considered whether to initially freeze embryos, we now look at the second consideration: What to do with unwanted frozen embryos.

Before doing IVF we asked ourselves, "What if we got seven embryos? Let's say we transferred three and froze four? What would we do if we got triplets on the first try? Would we actually go back and use the four remaining frozen embryos?" If not, we felt we shouldn't freeze. We were committed to all life that we created. Our lab made us sign papers stating what we'd do with frozen embryos if something hap- pened to us.

Certainly it is *more* ethical to thaw and transfer embryos than to dis- card some of the more than 400,000 frozen embryos that exist as of this writing. Half a chance is better than no chance.

Once a husband and wife agree to freeze embryos, they must face some additional choices: Will they store them for their own future use, donate them for research, let them be destroyed, or donate them to other infertile couples for adoption?

Respecting life at the one-cell stage means giving all embryos a chance to live rather than letting them thaw and die—which eliminates the options of research and destruction. Though it might sound noble to donate an embryo for the furtherance of science, the decision to do so would fail ethically. The destruction of human life violates beneficence, nonmaleficence, the embryo's personal autonomy, and justice. How is it "just" to destroy a life without its consent, even for the benefit of another?

To give every cryopreserved life a chance means having remaining frozen embryos thawed and transferred to the wife, donating them for adoption, or finding someone who will carry them to term.

Stop!

If we still have frozen embryos when our family is complete, should we do "compassionate transfer"?

Our doctor said he wanted to transfer only two embryos, and if we had twins and didn't want more children, he could do "compassionate transfer" of any remaining embryos. That is, he'd transfer them at a time in my cycle when I'm unlikely to get pregnant. Isn't that nearly the same as discarding? It is giving them a "chance," but hoping they won't make it. The doctor said he doesn't believe embryos are life until they implant and there's a heartbeat.

Clinic names for this type of technique vary, but the procedure was developed to soothe the consciences of those who have "extra" embryos and don't want to carry them to term or destroy them outright. The physician thaws and transfers the four-cell or six-cell (not blastocyst) embryo to the uterus without all the synchronizing hormones, aiming for transfer during a time when the uterus is unreceptive to pregnancy. This process has a near-zero success rate, though the embryo has a fractionally higher chance of living than if it were thawed and left in a dish. When considered in light of the construct, this is an unethical option.

Stop!

What are the ethics of donating embryos for research? The blastocyst has received considerable media attention in the debate about stem cell research for the possible cure of an assortment of diseases (diabetes, Parkinson's, spinal cord trauma).[8] Thus, many couples have considered donating their "excess" embryos for use in this research. The motivation behind such an altruistic act, while praiseworthy, has ethical implications.[9]

The blastocyst (early embryo) is made up of perhaps 100 to 200 cells that appear in a hollow, spherical shape with an additional cluster of cells inside one end. These inner cells represent the embryonic pole, the very cells forming the embryo. To harvest these inner cells (embryonic stem cells) for research, the embryo and the supportive cells must be destroyed. Thus, donating cryopreserved embryos for stem cell research actually means the thawing of an embryo to kill it. While this may soothe the consciences of the genetic parents, it fails each of the ethical parameters from the standpoint of the tiny human being. The innocent embryo is killed, clearly an injustice, without ever having a chance to express autonomy.

Embryonic stem cells *can* be obtained from unwanted frozen embryos. Thus, many people have distinguished in their minds a difference between therapeutic cloning (for medical research) and reproductive cloning (to produce a baby identical to its genetic parent). It is reasoned that because the embryos will not be transferred anyway, they may as well be used for research.

The creation of cloned human cell lines (cloned humans from which the embryonic stem cells are extracted and then guided to grow into a specific kind of cell) involves taking the genetic material from an adult cell (skin, muscle, or even mammary cells as first done in Dolly the sheep). That material is then placed into a human egg that has had its nucleus removed so you won't have two separate nuclei trying to run the show. This cloned cell is then stimulated with electrical current or a chemical solution to "switch on" all the proper cells for embryonic growth (*without,* presumably, "flipping any switches" that lead to abnormalities such as catastrophic birth defects or those causing cancer). The clone is allowed to divide up to the blastocyst stage. Then, rather than the blastocyst being transferred into an awaiting womb where pregnancy can continue (reproductive cloning), the embryonic cells are extracted, *killing the clone* (therapeutic cloning). The only thing preventing the therapeutic clone from becoming a reproductive clone is that with therapeutic cloning, the researcher intervenes and destroys the embryo rather than transferring it to the uterus. Reproductive cloning, though its goal is a new human life, still exceeds the limit of God-given dominion. It is immoral and is opposed almost universally.

Stop!

What about preimplantation genetic diagnosis? Preimplantation genetic diagnosis (PGD) is similar to standard prenatal testing, with two key differences: (1) testing for problems happens after fertilization in the IVF lab. Embryos are analyzed for more than one hundred genetic conditions, including Alzheimer's, fragile X syndrome, Down syndrome, Huntington's disease, hemophilia, and cystic fibrosis. PGD sex selection is also done to prevent gender-linked disorders. (2) All embryos found to be "defective" are destroyed.

PGD is also being used to improve live birthrates for women who have previously had unexplained, recurrent pregnancy losses. In one study, researchers noted that almost 70 percent of the embryos screened via PGD among women with recurrent pregnancy loss were abnormal, confirming the theory that chromosomal problems may be largely responsible for the recurrent losses.[10]

The procedure, developed in the 1990s, has resulted in at least 1,000 births of preselected embryos. The cost runs between $1,500 and $3,000, in addition to the cost of IVF. It is estimated that in the future, about 20 percent of IVF cycles will include PGD. One expert noted, "Most people are quite happy to use PGD to prevent serious life-damaging, painful, horrendous diseases. But do you do it to prevent diabetes? At what point is society willing to say it doesn't want an embryo to survive?"[11]

Clearly, infertility can be like a moral maze full of constant turns and decisions and dead ends. Knowing that, perhaps we should take a moment to redefine "success." Success, as far as God is concerned, is not ultimately about having the desired child. It's far greater than that. Success is living according to Scripture (Josh. 1:8). Biblical limits are not given to make life less enjoyable. Rather, the limits are like a map through a minefield, which prevents us from causing more damage.

Though about 35 percent of couples who go through infertility treatment will never experience successful pregnancies, all couples in treatment can make good decisions while holding fast to God and to each another. Each of us will one day account for our actions (Rom. 14:12). Those who make wise decisions during the process of treatment find that they are content and have no regrets long after their painful years of infertility treatment are behind them.

DISCUSSION QUESTIONS

1. Now that you have a construct through which to process ethical decisions, reconsider the answers you gave in chapter 13 in light of this information. Did anything change for you?

2. If no other technology were available for you, would you consider cloning to produce a child?

3. Consider your infertility workup to date. Has it proven to be ethical when viewed through the construct presented in this chapter?

4. Are you considering any current treatment approaches that may be over the line ethically? If so, what?

5. Do you and your spouse agree on these issues? If not, where do you disagree?

6. Do you and your medical team agree on these issues? If not, where do you disagree?

7. Have you discussed with your medical team each step of the workup and treatment plan? How might you take a more active role in the future?

8. How far is "too far" as you evaluate your treatment options with your ethical understanding?

Chapter 15

THREE'S COMPANY

THIRD-PARTY REPRODUCTION

In one infertility cartoon, an angry woman has wheeled a baby buggy carrying Mickey Mouse into a donor sperm clinic. The clinic director tells her, "Look lady, you're the one who asked for a famous movie star with dark hair, a strong nose, and deep-set eyes." Along those same lines, a story is told of George Bernard Shaw in the early 1900s. A beautiful opera singer approached him with, "We would have such beautiful babies, with my looks and your brains." Shaw, an intellectual, quipped, "But my dear, imagine if the child had my looks and your brains."[1]

Mention artificial insemination by donor, or "donor insemination" (DI)—the oldest and most widespread technique of assisted reproduction—and many people bristle. They make derogatory remarks about "designer babies," "custom-made children," "turkey-baster babies," "spiritual adultery," "adultery by doctor," or "sex with a syringe." And they might mention the Repository for Germinal Choice, the sperm bank where Nobel Prize winners supposedly send their sperm.[2]

Since the development of micromanipulation, couples increasingly opt for such in vitro fertilization (IVF) techniques rather than choosing DI. Yet despite this trend, DI is still the most commonly used artificial conception procedure worldwide. More than a million children have been born through DI.[3] Donor insemination works the same as husband insemination except instead of coming from the husband, sperm comes from a donor. Married couples choose DI for cases in which the husband has an untreatable condition—whether a sperm problem, a spinal-cord injury, a failed vasectomy reversal, or a genetic problem he could pass on.

- Thomas, a married tennis pro in his late thirties, produced no sperm. After months of deliberating, he and his wife chose to build their family by donor insemination (DI). Initially devastated by his diagnosis, Thomas said, "Once we made the decision, it was okay."

- The parents of two children having a Y-linked genetic disorder were told to try IVF with the option of testing the embryos, then transferring only the healthy ones. Because they believed disposing of any "unhealthy" embryos would be taking life, the doctor recommended donor insemination.

Rob, a pastor, was shocked when his semenalysis revealed no sperm. He said, "We tried donor insemination one time unsuccessfully. We probably could have achieved a pregnancy had we stayed with it, but we stopped. Our church members would've said, 'We prayed and Rob was healed!' It would have felt dishonest. If the truth had become known, many might have misunderstood or been offended. As a pastor, I feel a heightened responsibility to keep from causing a 'weaker brother'—that is a person who's less mature in the faith—to stumble. If we were not in a public ministry, I'm pretty sure we'd have gone for it."

The first recorded cases of human artificial insemination date back to the turn of the nineteenth century in England and France, following the discovery of the process of inseminating animals. This discovery was made by an abbot who did scientific experiments to determine whether life originated with the human egg or with sperm. [4] A Philadelphia doctor performed the first known successful DI technique in 1909. He didn't tell the husband until afterward, and then the two agreed never to tell the wife. Fortunately, today the trend is away from secrecy.

An FDA study estimated that 80,000 to 100,000 donor inseminations are performed in the United States each year. [5] The American market for donor sperm is conservatively estimated at $20 million dollars, and the United States is the biggest exporter of sperm in the world.

Clinics and sperm banks, of which there are about 150 in the United States, screen potential donors for health, fertility, and infectious diseases, including HIV and hepatitis, which can both survive the freeze-thaw process. Clinics and sperm banks also check for risky sexual practices and exposure to toxins and radiation. Men who produce less than 20 million sperm per sample are disqualified. According to one sperm bank, only about 3 to 5 percent of potential donors are accepted into their program.

Once collected, semen is typically cryopreserved for at least six months, during which time the donor is retested for infectious disease at regular intervals. Freezing decreases the sperm's fertility potential. Conceiving with frozen sperm takes an average of five menstrual cycles, compared with three cycles using fresh sperm. But freezing the sperm and then testing the donor before releasing his sample decreases the odds of passing on communicable diseases. Insemination is almost always done as intrauterine insemination (IUI), rather than vaginal insemination, to give sperm an additional advantage because of the decreased motility associated with the freeze-thaw process.

The congenital abnormality rates of offspring created using frozen sperm are the same as with fresh sperm inseminations (the same as in the general population).[6] Those most likely to conceive using DI are women under the age of thirty-five.

But scientific feasibility does not guarantee ethical acceptability. Just because we *can* do something does not mean we *should* do it. What about the ethics of third-party reproduction? Certainly, not all authorities agree.

We encourage couples considering donor insemination to explore two key elements in the equation: special revelation and general revelation. *Special revelation* relates to what God has directly decreed about himself and his ways. It includes stories and principles from the Bible that instruct us about how to live. We can also learn from creation and the world around us—*general revelation*. Jesus said, "Consider the lilies of the field, how they grow," so that we would observe what they reveal to us about God's care (Matt. 6:28 NKJV). An analysis of general revelation includes considering whatever data we have from the best research available.

Using these criteria, we will now explore such questions as, "Is third-party reproduction wise?" and "What right, if any, do children have to know about their genetic origins?" Both of us agree that our personal opinions have been crystallized through time, experience, and study. We see donor insemination as an issue of personal conviction, not a clear "sin" issue.

Special Revelation

Many Christian leaders have been quick to condemn DI. For example, a well-known Christian psychologist stated in his monthly national magazine that DI is always wrong, even if it involves a sibling donor. The speaker at a Christian bioethics conference noted how infertile couples "take a low view of God's gift of sex in favor of an inflated view of technology." The remark suggested that couples choose high-tech options over sexual intimacy as thrill-seeking attempts to surf on the edge of technology. The speaker went on to express that reproductive technologies reflect a devaluation of God's design for the beauty of sex in favor of something artificial.

Afterward an infertility patient confided, "Believe me, every infertile person I know would much rather conceive 'the natural way' over lying alone on a table in a doctor's office!"

Couples often willingly enter a complex maze of moral dilemmas in their quest for a biological child. Why? They recognize the value of a child, and that recognition sometimes presses them to skirt the edge of ethics because the end result is so precious.

God blessed the first couple with the opportunity to multiply and fill the earth. Picture Adam and Eve ready to create an entire race. They had no manuals, helps, doctors, or knowledge of temperature charting. Certainly, there was no option of a third party.

Most couples envision it will be as simple for them. They dream about producing together a child that's the product of their love—not the product of their love plus a physician, a lot of debt, invasive procedures, and maybe even a donor. Wrapped up in infertility lie unfulfilled longings and the death of precious dreams.

What does the Bible say that might inform our thinking about third-party reproduction? We begin by asking, "Would God ever allow a third party to enter a marriage arrangement?" It appears that he did.

Polygamy

Abraham and Jacob both had more than one wife. So did David, Solomon, and Gideon. In Genesis, we read that when Leah saw that she had stopped conceiving, she gave her maid Zilpah to her husband as a wife (Gen. 30:9). Later Leah went on to conceive a fifth son, and she named him Issachar, meaning "hire," or "wages." Her reasoning for naming him that? "*God* has given me my wages." Why? "*Because* I have given my maid to my husband" (v. 18 NASB, italics ours). Leah believed she had done the right thing and God had rewarded her.

After David committed adultery with Bathsheba, Nathan brought him a message from the Lord, including these words: "I gave your master's house to you, and your master's wives *into your arms*. I gave you the house of Israel and Judah. And if all this had been too little, I would have given you even more" (2 Sam. 12:8, italics ours). The Hebrew word for "arms" here is translated "lap" in the book of Ruth (4:16): "Then Naomi took the child, laid him in her *lap* and cared for him." Older translations say "bosom." God clearly gave Saul's former wives to David in what was to be more than a distant "financial support only" arrangement.

In Deuteronomy 21:15, the text says, "If a man has two wives, the one loved but not the other, and both bear him sons but the firstborn is the son of the wife he does not love, when he wills his property to his sons, he must not give the rights of the firstborn to the son of the wife he loves in preference to his actual firstborn."

We're not recommending the practice of polygamy or even suggesting that God preferred it then or approves of it today! The pain involved in such arrangements is recorded both in Scripture (consider Sarah and Hagar, Rachel and Leah, Hannah and Peninnah) and in many case studies. In societies today that practice polygamy, the wives in such arrangements often share the injustice and emotional pain they suffer. Through God's continuing revelation, we see redemptive movement away from polygamy and toward a one-flesh ideal (Eph. 5:31). By the time of the New Testament, the practice of having multiple wives was unacceptable for godly people.[7] Our point here is only to demonstrate that those who say "God has never allowed a third party into a marriage" will have difficulty making their case based on the scriptural evidence.

Levirate Marriage

Another example of a marriage involving a third party to produce a child is in the case of levirate marriage (Deut. 25:5–6). In the book of Ruth, we see this practice, in which a surviving brother (or a near relative, as was the case with Boaz and Ruth) took his sister-in-law as his wife to give the deceased brother an heir. The firstborn child from their union carried the family name of the deceased. This practice sometimes involved polygamy if the man was already married.[8] Interestingly, when polygamy was abolished in the ancient Near East—over a thousand years ago—Jewish law determined that the command to practice levirate marriage should also no longer be practiced.[9] Apparently, levirate marriage and polygamy were frequently linked. While we have nothing like levirate marriage in the West, in some cultures, such as tribal groups in Zambia, it is still practiced. And in the Old Testament, God commanded it. He even killed Onan (Gen. 38:10) for refusing to care for his brother's widow in this way. While we would like to believe that only unmarried brothers took their widowed sisters-in-law as wives, polygamy was probably sometimes involved.

As should be obvious from these texts, levirate marriage provides "biblical precedent for third-party involvement."[10] Nevertheless, while a few biblical scholars have pointed to such arrangements as the earliest form of donor insemination, there are actually some obvious differences between the two. First, the widow *married* the "donor," even if it meant polygamy. Second, the biological father was not anonymous, as is often the case with modern donors. Third, the children had a deep connection to their roots and thus had strong identities within their genetic families. Many adult donor offspring today deeply grieve their disconnection from their genetic roots. In fact, many donor offspring suffer a state of confusion known as "genealogical bewilderment" when deprived of this information. And fourth, God allowed third-party reproduction in a culture in which infertility meant more than just the longing for a child. Sometimes infertility meant the couple's very survival was threatened. There would be no children to care for the couple in their old age. Hospitals and nursing homes did not exist, so the responsibility for aging parents fell on the children. In case of third-party reproduction, there was nothing secretive, anonymous, or impersonal about the genetic father. And there were no fees or forms from doctors or attorneys—a definite plus!

Some people have wondered whether, based on the levirate picture, using a close relative as a donor might somehow provide a donor in the spirit of levirate marriage. But there's a key difference between the two. With levirate marriage, the first husband was dead, so there was only one father in the equation. With a relative donor, two men would share an affinity with the child. Thus, a rabbinical student raises some important questions for the donor in such a case: "Will you be able to look at the child as your nephew, rather than your son? What if the child was told, or found out later, that you were his biological father, and wanted a different relationship with you? What if your brother and his wife divorced or your brother died? What if you felt the child was ill-treated? What if you and your future wife were unable to have children? . . . While your brother is now grateful for your help, later on, he may resent your ability to have fathered the child he could not."[11]

In all of the biblical examples, the biological father of the child actually parented the child. A modern donor does not.

The One-Flesh Principle

At one time in my medical practice, I (Dr. Bill) did inseminations for patients using donor sperm. I never knew of patients who had legal problems or major complications—unless you count the woman who told me that while she sat in my waiting area, she watched for unusual men coming and going, wondering, "Is *he* our donor?" Seeing one particularly unsavory fellow motivated her to ask me pleadingly, "Is it *him*?" (It wasn't.)

Eventually I limited inseminations to only those using the husband's sperm. This was, for me, a matter of prayerful conviction. A friend, colleague, and brother in Christ sees it differently. Joe McIlhaney, M.D., a committed Christian and a good thinker who has served for years on the board of Focus on the Family, says the following in his book *Dear*

God, Why Can't We Have a Baby? "Donor inseminations have been part of my infertility practice for many years. I have prayerfully considered the biblical, moral and ethical aspects of this procedure and am comfortable performing it. . . . It might interest couples who feel [DI] is right for them to know that I have not had any couple express any regret about having undergone the [DI] procedure. Several couples have returned to have a second child using [DI]. Many of these women are long-term patients and I am not aware of any problems that developed for them or their husbands after using [DI] to help them have a child."

My decision to use only a husband's sperm came after much soul searching. It is based on what I refer to as the "one flesh" guideline. Although we do see a few similarities to third-party situations in the biblical text, perhaps this one-flesh principle can offer us a more helpful guide in decision making when we approach rapidly advancing medical technology. The Bible describes marriage as "two become one," a picture of intimacy and unity. The marriage bond is sacred, a covenant between two people before God that no one should tear apart. Applying this one-flesh exclusivity, we would conclude that any technology allowing the husband-wife union to produce children is acceptable assuming no other laws of God (such as the sanctity of life) are violated as part of the procedure. In other words, the one-flesh guideline means any technology that enables the husband and wife to produce a child using their own gametes (eggs, sperm) is acceptable as long as the sanctity of human life is upheld. It would also allow for adoption of existing embryos whose gametes come from neither husband nor wife.

I want to emphasize that this is my personal guideline, which appears to me consistent with Scripture, and *not* the clear teaching of Scripture, making all other positions erroneous or worse! Nevertheless, I have found it helpful. Using this one-flesh guideline, any technology that mixes the gametes of a third party with one of the spouse's gametes would be unacceptable. Thus, I would condone the following:

- artificial insemination using the husband's sperm.
- in vitro fertilization using the husband's and wife's sperm and eggs, assuming the embryo is treated with respect.
- embryo adoption and its associated gestational surrogacy (more on this in chapter 16).

Some have suggested that "they [the two] shall become one flesh" (Gen. 2:24 NASB) is a reference only to the marital sexual union, but it's broader than that.[12] Others have suggested that it's a physical and emotional oneness, and while that is certainly involved, it would appear this interpretation is still too narrow. Genesis seems to be talking about how husband and wife become relatives in a mysterious way by God's involvement—whether or not they acknowledge him. In saying this, we recognize that this passage is not referring to reproductive technologies, nor does it even give a principle for handling reproductive technologies. Yet it does refer to an exclusiveness in the husband-wife relationship, the spirit of which, in my humble opinion, is broad enough to encompass this issue.

It's also important to note here that mercy is always appropriate. Perhaps if more people considered the unusual practices that were allowed for overcoming infertility in biblical times (polygamy, concubines), they might be slower to criticize infertile couples who try high-tech methods. While some have read the Bible's emphasis on alternatives for childbearing and interpreted them as presenting a cruel overemphasis on reproduction, one could also read the same passages and see a great deal of flexibility allowed for fulfilling such deep longings (Prov. 30:15–16). There is a degree of creativity in how God allowed families to be built in times past.

Spiritual Adultery?

One clear difference between today's practices and those in biblical times is that modern third-party arrangements do not involve a physical relationship between a spouse and the donor. Some have minimized this difference by using inflammatory language to refer to donor insemination as "spiritual adultery."

One infertile husband wrote, "I believe that artificial inseminations with donor semen are a form of adultery.... Donor insemination amounts to technical adultery, because you take the semen of a man not the wife's husband and use it to conceive.... The use of sperm banks, surrogate mothers, and illegal adoptions are surely not acceptable for the mature Christian trying to do God's will."[13]

Clearly, the Bible speaks strongly against adultery, but in what sense is DI a violation of "You shall not commit adultery"? Adultery involves sexual intercourse. Jesus further amplified the definition of adultery by stating that to "look at a woman lustfully" was to commit adultery in one's heart (Matt. 5:28).

As stated earlier, I performed many donor inseminations during my early years of practice, and I am familiar with the process of donor selection, specimen preparation, and insemination. There is no physical contact between the donor and the recipient, and often no exchange of identifying information. Certainly, there is no lust on the part of the recipient. Thus, adultery is not involved in the process of DI.

Interestingly, though today's Jewish law does not permit DI, most rabbinic authorities say that DI should not be considered adultery. Thus, a child born by donor insemination is not illegitimate.[14]

If we are going to object to third-party scenarios, let's at least do so for the right reasons.

As we have tried to demonstrate, in considering third-party reproduction, the first step for the earnest believer is to explore the spiritual ramifications. One pastor describes the process that he and his wife went through: "We prayed and asked God for healing, which he chose not to do. After getting a realistic picture of adoption, we considered alternatives. We were counseled toward DI by one of our specialists. In working through the moral, ethical, and spiritual issues, we prayed, studied Scriptures, talked to elders and other pastors." We encourage our readers faced with third-party reproduction to consider the spiritual and ethical ramifications as deeply as they consider the medical possibilities.

DISCUSSION QUESTIONS

1. Have you given thought to third-party issues? If so, what have you concluded?
2. Do you see third-party reproduction as an option for you? For others you know?
3. Do you consider third-party reproduction a wisdom issue, a fidelity issue, and/or a theological issue?
4. How would you feel either to receive donor gametes or for your partner to do so?
5. If you oppose DI, we encourage you to do so for the right reasons. What might be some invalid reasons for saying DI is wrong? What are the stronger arguments?

Chapter 16

AID IN THE BEGETTING

DONOR EGG, SURROGACY, AND EMBRYO ADOPTION

Donor Egg (DE)

[Donor egg] is a wonderful option, and I thank God that it's available because it's my only hope to have a child. I just can't help but feel sad because my dad passed away unexpectedly and I'd have loved to have had a child with a little part of Dad mixed in. He was a caring and wonderful man. If he were still here, he would have encouraged me and would have loved our child just as much, genetic link or not. I know in my heart that if I am lucky enough to succeed in having a baby that I will still look for any similarities.

I've struggled with the loss of the genetic link, but the following thinking helps: If DE succeeds, we'll overcome 2.5 out of 3 losses—1 is the fulfillment of my desire to parent; 2 is experiencing pregnancy and childbirth; 3 is genetic continuity. With DE I get the first two and half of the three—our child will have my husband's genes.

Our longing to have a child is stronger than the obstacles of using an egg donor. We both have great careers, but a job isn't everything. Having a child leaves a more enduring legacy than what we do at our jobs.

A husband and wife hover over a computer screen, clicking until they land on a site that says, "Our services include open, semiopen, or anonymous recipient-donor relationships." They start looking for a "good match," scanning through pictures of beautiful, educated women between the ages of nineteen and thirty-two.[1] Each candidate has been screened for excellent health and freedom from sexually transmitted diseases.

There's Mara, the twenty-three-year-old Olympic gold medalist, but she wants $50,000 for one cycles' worth of her eggs. Then there's Laura, a twenty-year-old blonde at Princeton, who has a 3.5 grade point average. She's asking only $25,000. The most affordable is Stephanie at Yale. Her price: $20,000.

The husband and wife sigh and move to another site where the candidates have less glamorous resumes but physical and mental characteristics that more closely match the wife's, and a price tag that is more reasonable. It frustrates the couple that between 1998 and 2002, the going rate for a woman's eggs tripled. So many patients seek donors that clinics, in a competitive market, respond to the demand by offering donors more money. The infertile couple pays the price. And price is the name of the game.

Cost. Compared with donor insemination, conceiving with donor eggs is extremely expensive. Many clinics require recipient couples to buy insurance policies for the donor through the clinic. Such policies, generally not sold to individuals, cost hundreds of dollars per cycle. And that's before the cycle begins.

When it comes to the cycle itself, the egg donor goes through the in vitro fertilization (IVF) process of ovulation stimulation and egg harvest. Because the couple's insurance won't cover her medical costs, they must pay for the procedure. At the time of this writing, it is estimated that DE costs about $30,000. The couple mentioned above doesn't begrudge the amount charged by women for "donor reimbursement" in the under-$5,000 range recommended by the ethics committee of the American Society for Reproductive Medicine (ASRM). The couple believes the donor deserves some compensation for the grueling process she'll experience. Unlike sperm donors, whose "contribution" takes only a few minutes of minimal physical exertion followed by an endorphin rush, egg donors endure weeks of shots and medical procedures, with no roses and no pleasure.

Screening. Because the process is so involved, some clinics have shut down their DE programs for lack of donors. And some clinics overuse donors, allowing them to donate for up to ten cycles. But most clinics limit this number to two cycles. Most donors report feeling proud, viewing their donation one of the most important acts they have ever done. So far, according to one clinic that has interviewed 800 donors, donors' postdonation concerns tend to focus less on their genetic children and more on possible long-term negative effects of the medications. At this point, we don't know the long-term effect DE has on the healthy donors' own fertility and egg supplies.

Many clinics encourage couples to recruit their own donors. And unlike with donor insemination (DI), the wait for a donor may be a long one. It has been estimated that it takes about five months to go through the donor selection process, and many clinics have a waiting list of a year or more. Couples may work through a variety of sources to find their own donors—a clinic, a donor-egg broker, internet contacts, family, friends, and advertisements.

Clinics screen egg donors for the same things they look for with sperm donors. Yet because the month-long process of ovulation induction is so much more rigorous, screening often includes psychological assessment. Scientists who examined the mental states of 607 women who volunteered to become egg donors found that 11 percent of them "had psychological findings that prohibited them from participating." Most of the rejected donors had personal histories of mental illness, learning disabilities, alcohol or substance abuse, or criminal records, while others had family histories of these characteristics or a family history of suicide.[2]

The physical process a donor must go through is challenging, basically paralleling IVF. (DE does have a higher success rate than traditional IVF, however, due to the younger age of the eggs.) While the average number of eggs harvested per retrieval runs between eight and ten, it can vary between zero (rare) and forty (also rare). A high number of eggs usually means a greater number of immature eggs, so sometimes less is more.

Success and failure. In DE procedures, a donor's eggs are fertilized with sperm, usually from the recipient's husband, and transferred to the wife or a gestational surrogate, whose menstrual cycle has been synchronized with the donor's. The baby has five potential "parents" in this process—a sperm donor, an egg donor, a surrogate, and the two adoptive parents!

Eighty-five percent of the time, fertilization of at least one egg will happen. Fertilization is considered successful if 60 to 70 percent of the eggs fertilize. (With a high number of eggs, the number achieving fertilization may be lower, around 50 percent.) In cases with no fertilization, the couple must still pay all the costs for the attempt. Implantation rates tend to be lower when an especially high number of eggs are retrieved. Sometimes clinics do assisted hatching on the embryos before transfer to aid implantation.

If the first cycle fails to result in pregnancy, some clinics do blastocyst transfer (BT), as outlined in chapter 12. Early studies suggest this may aid implantation, but it's still under investigation.

While artificial insemination using donor sperm has been around for more than a hundred years, the option of using a donor egg didn't exist until 1984. Now as we see an increasing number of couples choosing micromanipulation over DI, we see more women using donor eggs to overcome the effects of aging. The donor-egg industry has been growing rapidly as new studies show that the chance of having a baby is the same for women in their forties as it is for women in their twenties if the egg donor is under thirty.[3]

Candidates. Counselors describe a variety of typical snapshots of families seeking an egg donor. The most frequent picture they see is a couple in their forties with secondary infertility. Another is the couple that has adopted in the past and would like to give their child a sibling. In this case, the wife still longs to experience pregnancy and give birth. Naturally, these are not the only scenarios, but they are among the most common.

Most women using egg donors are premenopausal. About 250 women age fifty or older gave birth in 2000, according to the National Center for Health Statistics, up from 160 in 1960. Only a few dozen women are known to have had babies at age fifty-five or older, though those numbers are likely to increase. (The Centers for Disease Control does not keep statistics on birthrates for women over fifty-four.)

Couples use donor eggs in a variety of medical situations: ovarian failure in women under forty years old; absence of ovaries due to congenital problems, cancer, endometriosis, or pelvic infection; repeated IVF failure because of poor egg or embryo quality; damaged ovaries due to cancer treatment; natural menopause; and to avoid transmitting genetic disease.

Fresh or frozen? Slightly more than 11 percent of ART cycles done in the year 2001 involved couples using donated eggs or embryos. Of those, less than one-third used frozen donor gametes; most used fresh gametes. Whereas frozen specimens are usually used in procedures involving sperm donation, the freeze-thaw process with eggs is not nearly as efficient, so most clinics use fresh eggs.

The morality of DE according to special revelation. To determine whether couples should pursue conceiving via egg donor, we use the same process as with sperm donation—looking at special and general revelation. We've already explored what the biblical record (special revelation) suggests to us about third-party reproduction. Additionally, a large number of Jewish, Islamic, Protestant, and Roman Catholic authorities condemn the use of donor gametes. Consider this statement by the Vatican:

Respect for the unity of marriage and for conjugal fidelity demands that the child be conceived in marriage; the bond existing between husband and wife accords the spouses, in an objective and inalienable manner, the exclusive right to become father and mother solely through each other. Recourse to the gametes of the third person in order to have sperm or ovum available constitutes a violation of the reciprocal commitment of the spouses and a grave lack in regard to the essential property of marriage which is its unity.

[Third-party reproduction] violates the rights of the child: It deprives him of his filial relationship with his parental origins and can hinder the maturity of his personal identity. Consequently, fertilization of a married woman with the sperm of a donor different from her husband and fertilization with the husband's sperm of an ovum not coming from his wife are morally illicit.[4]

The Christian Medical and Dental Associations came to a similar determination about donor gametes: "Clinical IVF and embryo transfer is justified morally only within the context of the marital bond, using 'gametes obtained from lawfully married couples' as the recommendations of the Ethics Advisory Board of the Department of Health, Education and Welfare have indicated."[5]

The morality of DE according to general revelation. What can we learn about the morality of using a donor by observing the world around us? So far, egg donation has not been around long enough for the offspring to share their feelings about it, but we suspect that the issues parallel many of the issues associated with DI.

An internet survey of DE recipient couples found that with sperm donation, women were more willing than men to tell their children about the donor. We might expect to see the reverse with egg donation, but we don't. Women in families built by egg donation are still more likely than their husbands to tell others that they used donor eggs. One study with 236 participants found the following:

- 80 percent of the women and 50 percent of the men had told at least one other person.
- Two-thirds of the women and 79 percent of the men studied said that faced with the same choice again, they would withhold the information.[6]
- Another study found that in egg donor families, 8 percent of the women and 5 percent of the men had already told the child. (Keep in mind the relative newness of DE and the young age of the offspring.)

- 39 percent of the women and 60 percent of the men had no intentions of ever telling the child, while half of the women and a fourth of the men did plan to tell the child.
- More than 90 percent reported that they had obtained medical information about the egg donor, and 10 percent had wanted to see a photo.[7]

Regardless of whether a couple elects disclosure or nondisclosure, it is vital that both husband and wife have the same attitudes about the degree of openness desired. Little research or even anecdotal evidence is available about the feelings of egg-donor offspring because it is still such a relatively new option. However, the parents of donor-conceived twins (now in the fifth grade) wrote this:

We believe it's crucial that we inform our children about how they were conceived—through egg donation. First, they have a right to know. Second, keeping secrets can be damaging. Our daughter wants to see what the donor looks like and if she has kids, but we've told her that's impossible—we made a promise.

In addition to the feelings of offspring, it is interesting also to note the feelings donors have in retrospect. One study revealed the following:

- 44 percent were "very satisfied" with their donation experience.
- 37 percent would be unwilling to donate again.
- 35 percent would be willing to donate again.
- 28 percent were not certain either way.

Compensation turned out to be a factor in their decision-making process. All of the women felt that donors should receive some financial compensation for their effort, though 77 percent also said the act of helping another woman was an important motivation for becoming an egg donor.

- 44 percent of the women had received $5,000.
- 16 percent received $3,500.
- 16 percent received $3,000.
- 23 percent received $2,000–$2,500.

Only 11 percent said they would be willing to donate without compensation.[8]

Surrogacy

Surrogacy presents additional factors that couples must consider. A couple must appoint a guardian for the child in the event of their deaths or incapacitations during the time when the surrogate is carrying their child. And there is the question of how many embryos to transfer. If the surrogate conceives, is she willing to carry triplets? Where does she stand on selective reduction?

Let's consider the two types of surrogacy arrangements: traditional and gestational.

Traditional surrogacy. Traditional surrogacy (via artificial insemination) is generally used when a pregnancy would be life-threatening for the mother or when a patient has neither functioning ovaries nor a uterus. The surrogate's own eggs are fertilized with the sperm of the husband by artificial insemination. She then carries the pregnancy to term. Traditional surrogacy carries with it more complicated issues than do sperm and egg donation or embryo adoption, because in a surrogate arrangement, the surrogate-donor has contact with the child through the nine-month gestation and the birth, and she has both a biological and a genetic connection to the child. After the birth, the surrogate relinquishes parental rights, and the client husband and wife become the child's legal parents.

One of the disadvantages of such an arrangement is that it has the potential to negatively impact the marriage relationship. This risk is even greater with traditional surrogacy than with DI. Rather than dropping off a "gamete sample," the donor in this case enters a relationship in which she conceives the husband's baby, has a nine-month pregnancy, and then delivers. In the best scenario, the couple is actively involved with her throughout the pregnancy.

With traditional surrogacy, the "bypassed" parent has much more potential to feel like an outsider as she watches another woman bear her husband's child. As one woman explained it: "We considered surrogacy. We asked my sister and she said yes, but her hubby would not agree. But it's hard enough just to see another woman pregnant right now. I can't imagine seeing someone else pregnant with our child."

Gestational surrogacy (via IVF). Gestational surrogacy involves a "host uterus" for a child that is genetically unrelated to the "gestational carrier," the woman in whose uterus the child is carried to term. The embryo comes from either the infertile couple's gametes fertilized in vitro, an embryo from the husband and an egg donor fertilized in vitro, or an adopted embryo from gametes of a different couple. The surrogate mother carries the child in utero, but she has no genetic link to it. In the case of a couple having their embryo transferred to a surrogate, the client family petitions the court to change the birth certificate to reflect the child's true genetic parentage. A gestational carrier is involved in only 1 percent of IVF cycles.

I want a biological child. I want to present my husband with our baby. It seems too unfair to him that I can't have children when he could be a biological father if he married someone else. We think that I make eggs and he has sperm, so why can't someone else carry the child? But is that ethical? How far can you go and still be within moral limits?

Both kinds of surrogacy have legal and moral ramifications, so couples pursuing these arrangements need to familiarize themselves with the laws, as they vary from state to state.

While one woman may have an intact uterus and thus need only an egg, another may have the opposite problem. A woman whose ovaries work fine but who has no uterus—or at least not a working one—may be told to consider a surrogate.

More than a quarter-century has passed since the first U.S. commercial surrogate birth in the late 1970s. But most people think of surrogacy as having a much longer history than that. Isn't surrogacy what Abraham and Sarah tried with Hagar, which caused all sorts of problems? Not exactly. For one thing, today's fertilization process is far less intimate than Abraham's relationship with Hagar. And today's surrogate doesn't move in as a cowife. She usually doesn't raise the child, either—unless something disastrous happens in the legal process.

Millennia after Abraham and Sarah's third-party arrangement, surrogacy has been providing plenty of media stories. We've seen the gutwrenching battle for "Baby M" when Mary Beth Whitehead changed her mind in 1985; we've witnessed the fifty-two-year-old Cheryl Tiegs announcing the birth of twin boys by a surrogate in 1990; and we've watched as Joan Lunden and her husband had twins via a surrogate mother. An estimated 16,000 babies have been born to surrogate mothers. (The exact number isn't known because many such arrangements take place between friends and family without documentation.)

Bring up the topic of surrogacy and most people, speaking of "wombs for rent," bring up these high-profile moms, nightmare court cases, and convoluted family structures. While we read tabloid stories about surrogates choosing to keep their babies, a surrogate often worries about the adoptive couple changing their minds and leaving her to raise a child or children that she's unprepared to handle. Consider the case of the couple who walked away from their surrogate because she conceived twins, and they wanted only one baby.[9]

Profile of a surrogate. Many people are surprised to learn that most surrogate mothers are married. The typical candidate has at least one child and is between twenty-five and thirty-five years old. These women have often had elective abortions and volunteer to bear a child as a means of healing from past decisions. Many surrogacy programs require that surrogates be finished bearing their own children before they agree to such arrangements.

Cost. Some centers estimate surrogacy costs between $35,000 and $50,000. Most of the money goes to someone other than the surrogate, such as the counselors, physicians, and attorneys who present clients with lengthy contracts. The traditional surrogate currently makes approximately $15,000 per pregnancy, plus $3,000 per extra child in multiple births. Gestational surrogacy (involving only a host uterus and not the surrogate's egg) is usually several thousand dollars less. This money is not for selling a full-term child but for taking the risks associated with a pregnancy, undergoing medical tests and procedures, and submitting to psychological testing and background checks. For the surrogate, this is a fifteen-month process that involves applying, being matched, carrying the child, and recovering.

Ethical considerations. In the past, most Christians—including the Christian Medical and Dental Associations[10]—have strongly opposed third-party arrangements, and in most cases they continue to do so. Yet when faced with the fact that many frozen embryos would otherwise be destroyed, infertile couples have sought the higher good. In those rare cases in which embryos are already frozen and the genetic mother is later rendered incapable of gestation, gestational surrogacy may be a permissible solution to an existing, undesirable ethical dilemma.

Such was the case for one Christian couple we met. They had done an IVF cycle during which multiple eggs were retrieved and six were fertilized. Three embryos were then placed in the wife's uterus, and the remaining three were cryopreserved. The wife went on to give birth, but medical complications required doctors to remove her uterus at the time of delivery. That left the couple with three frozen embryos and no means of carrying them. Because of their belief that each embryo is a precious, live human, they felt the right thing to do was to find someone who would help them carry the embryos to term. They wanted to raise their own genetic children rather than pursuing an embryo adoption arrangement, in which the gestational mother would keep the babies. So they spent $50,000—including legal, screening, and counseling fees—for a gestational carrier. Three embryos were transferred to the surrogate's uterus, and she give birth to twins.

Embryo Adoption

Another emerging option that involves a third-party arrangement, particularly among those who view each embryo as a precious life, is embryo adoption.

I was shocked when our doctor aspirated thirty-three eggs from my ovaries and fertilized all of them, producing more humans than I would ever be able to raise.

[Our daughter's] genetic parents chose us for embryo adoption the same way a birth mother chooses a family with whom she wants to place her child.

The whole procedure of embryo adoption was very positive. Whatever happened that went wrong in the past, we got it right this time. The baby was born healthy, and that's really the outcome we wanted—a happy, healthy baby.

Les and Candi had been trying to conceive for four years. Eventually they learned that Les was sterile and no surgical options could help his situation. Candi appeared to be fertile. They didn't want to try donor insemination because their spiritual beliefs made them uncomfortable with that option. Then they heard about the 400,000 embryos that sat frozen, at least 20,000 of which were slated for destruction unless someone was willing to carry them to term.[11] They realized that through embryo adoption, they could solve two problems: their inability to have a child and the needless destruction of a human being.

Embryo adoption appealed to Les and Candi because it would be giving a life a chance, preventing an otherwise pointless human death. So they contacted an embryo adoption program. They went through a process that included having a home study done and signing legal contracts. Before long, they were matched with a genetic family that wanted to place their thirteen embryos:

We saw six doctors, all of whom tried to discourage us from [embryo adoption]. Several doctors told us they would not work with us because they wanted us to try the simplest option (DI) first. Finally we found one doctor who agreed. But then he pressured us to transfer four embryos. We wanted to transfer only two but compromised on three. After the first transfer, I didn't conceive. The following month, three more were transferred—again unsuccessfully. Later we moved and found a new doctor, but his clinic uses blastocyst transfers. We struggled with that decision and are still unsure about it, but we had seven embryos left, and by the day of transfer, only one had survived. We transferred that one—and it worked. I'm due next month.

Surprisingly, 90 percent of couples who produce "surplus" frozen embryos through IVF prefer to have them destroyed rather than adopted by other infertile couples. Reasons for this include genetic parents wanting to avoid having their children brought up in other families—especially if the couple never successfully carried a pregnancy to term—as well as concerns about having siblings separated and about unwitting incest.[12] Because so few couples opt for making their embryos available for adoption, despite the fact that there are so many thousands of frozen embryos, demand for donated embryos still outstrips supply.

In the 1990s it was established that a 50 percent embryo thaw-survival rate was considered reasonable.[13] Today some clinics report that "about 70 percent of good quality embryos survive the thaw," but one has to wonder what percentage of live embryos did not qualify as "good quality" in the first place and were destroyed. As one clinic reports on their website, "From experience, two clear facts have emerged: (1) only the best embryos can withstand the trauma of the freeze-thaw process and (2) poor quality embryos tend to degenerate upon thawing. Our policy is only to freeze surplus embryos that are at least grade 3 or 4. These are embryos with even-sized cells and hardly any fragmentation."[14] This means some embryos, though still technically alive, are discarded because they are of "lesser quality." And some embryos that are of poor quality after the thaw are not transferred. And even if they are transferred, not all implant in the uterus.[15] Clearly, cryopreservation is traumatic to the embryo. In addition, there appears to be an increased risk of ectopic pregnancy with embryos that have been frozen.[16] Yet once an embryo has been frozen, the ethical solution is to thaw and transfer it (see chapter 14).

The process. Embryo adoption involves taking cryopreserved embryos that the genetic parents—for whatever reason—do not plan to transfer and matching those embryos with an adoptive couple.[17] (This is profoundly different from *embryo creation*—a process in which a couple selects both female and male donors based on intellect, ethnicity, and other physical features.)

Couples wishing to pursue embryo adoption can network to find their own donors or go through an agency. *Agency embryo adoption* involves an intermediating organization that works to match couples wishing to place their embryos with couples wanting to carry and raise them. Donating couples may select adoptive parents such as Les and Candi, who have passed a rigorous investigative process. The agency Les and Candi used has found that the genetic parents donating embryos to the agency tend to want their embryos to be born and raised in religious homes.[18]

Nonagency embryo adoption involves either a clinic making placements of embryos they have frozen or donors and recipients connecting independently and working out the details themselves. If genetic parents have expressed a desire to donate embryos and a clinic provides these embryos to another couple without the involvement of a psychological screening, matching, and home study process, it's often called *embryo donation*. With embryo donation, typically there is no contact between the two couples, even through an intermediary, and identities remain anonymous.

Once the adoptive couple has received frozen embryos, they are thawed and transferred to the uterus of the gestational mother, who will carry them to term. With embryo adoption, the arrangements may be open (identities are fully know), semiopen (some limited contact, some anonymity in details), or closed (full anonymity).

The first adopted embryo to complete gestation was born June 1998. Currently there are no laws governing embryo adoption, and at the time of this writing, about fifty babies had been born as a result of formal embryo adoption. (No verifiable figures exist on how many have been placed through anonymous or private embryo donation.) But demand is increasing, especially among infertile Christian couples. Typical candidates include women without ovaries, women at the older end of childbearing years, women with ovarian problems, couples with known genetic issues they don't want passed on, and couples in which the husband is sterile or has severe fertility problems.

While fertility treatments can cost up to $100,000 (depending on the number of IVF cycles couples do), and adoption can cost more than $10,000, agency embryo adoption costs about $6,000. (This includes legal fees and transport costs. It excludes the physicians' charge for embryo transfer.) Though it's far less expensive for couples to connect through a clinic or on the internet, adoption programs that require counseling and comprehensive testing are recommended. It is also recommended that both families involved in embryo adoption come to an agreement about confidentiality decisions, future contact questions, and what the child will be told. Some attorneys also recommend that couples ask the courts to recognize the genetic parents' contribution.

Many who are advocating embryo adoption are seeking to provide a solution to a problem: the potential destruction of human life. We hope that as people become aware of this option before they begin IVF, they will choose to limit the number of embryos created during their treatments to avoid creating a surplus. And anyone choosing to cryopreserve embryos should have a signed document on file both with their clinic and with their estate planner stating that, should they die, they desire for those embryos to be carried to term rather than destroyed. Couples should not treat casually the creation of "excess" embryos. They must avoid approaching IVF thinking, "We can do embryo adoption if we end up with more than we need." The actual decision to donate one's embryos for adoption is heart-wrenching.

Embryo adoption is an ethical solution to a less-than-ideal situation. But it's not without its problems. Therapists have raised some associated concerns that deserve consideration. The offspring will be the first group of children in history who were wanted but, because an embryologist chose their siblings for transfer to the genetic mother, were "deselected." When these offspring grow up, those in identified adoption situations may resent that their siblings live with the genetic parents they never got to know. And the siblings in the original family group may experience "survivor guilt." Beyond that, the genetic parents may wonder what life would have been like had they been able to keep their entire genetic family together.

Nevertheless, the ethics scale tips in favor of embryo adoption over destruction (it is better to save a life than to allow one to be destroyed), if the choice comes down to that.

- Does embryo adoption *"do good"*? Yes, the goal is to save a life and to treat a human with dignity and the full rights of personhood (Exod. 20:13).
- Does it *"do no harm"*? For the 50 percent that survive the thawing process, embryo adoption prevents harm from coming to the embryo (Matt. 25:40).
- Does it allow for patient *autonomy?* Since the embryo cannot speak for itself, a choice is made that is in the embryo's best interest (Prov. 31:8).
- Is it *just?* In embryo adoption, the embryo is treated as justly as is possible under the circumstances (Luke 6:31).

While the Roman Catholic Church opposes reproductive technologies in general, the Vatican statement affirms the goal of embryo adoption over donating embryos to research or destroying them: "As with all medical interventions on patients, one must uphold as licit [those] procedures carried out on the human embryo which respect the life and integrity of the embryo and do not involve disproportionate risks for it, but are directed toward its healing, the improvement of its condition of health or its individual survival."[19]

Why adopt embryos? The list of reasons for pursuing embryo adoption—such as wanting to experience the gestation and birth experiences—seems to be identical to reasons for doing other forms of third-party reproduction (see chapter 17). In fact, some clinics, failing to understand what drives couples to choose embryo donation over gamete donation try to steer them toward the latter option, as did Les and Candi's doctor. Clinic personnel may even go so far as to recommend embryo creation using donor eggs and sperm, oblivious to how much this suggestion bothers their patients.

The couples most likely to pursue embryo adoption frequently oppose using donor gametes. Often their underlying motivation (in addition to wanting a child) is that they value the sanctity of human life, even at the one-cell stage. They may see themselves as offering a solution to their own infertility that prevents the destruction of a human life. Their infertility has led them to allow a child to live who otherwise probably would have died.

Donating couples also view embryo adoption as a way to save their children's lives—to avoid human wastage of their own offspring. "We wanted to give them the best possible life and the best possible future," explains one genetic mother. "And that meant finding the right family for them."

Frozen donor embryo transfers represent a small percentage of ART cycles performed. The success rates for frozen donor embryos (27.3 percent per transfer) are lower than for fresh donor embryo transfers (47 percent).

How successful is frozen embryo transfer in nondonor situations? The 2001 data supports a 23.4 percent live birthrate per transfer[20] compared with 33.4 percent per transfer for fresh embryos.[21]

The providers for embryo adoption are often older than the average egg donors, and the freeze-thaw process appears to be hard on the embryo. But embryos stored for up to twelve years have been carried to term.[22] In most clinics, the best-quality embryos get used in the initial IVF cycle, and the rest are frozen for future use.

An embryo is a life that deserves a chance to be born. Today, through embryo adoption, tiny humans slated for destruction can become part of the solution to infertility for thousands of couples. As the mother of the first child born through embryo adoption said, "They're little boys and little girls, and God knows each one of them. . . . You tell me what I added to my daughter to make a human life."

DISCUSSION QUESTIONS

1. Do you feel that you have a complete understanding of the risks and benefits of the procedures covered in this chapter? If not, what do you need to do to become more informed?
2. What options have you explored as you've considered ways to resolve your infertility?
3. How much time do you think is needed to make such decisions?
4. Have you sought trained counsel? How might you benefit from counsel?
5. Do you believe secrets are always lethal? How would you handle disclosure issues? If you were to use an anonymous donor versus an identified donor, how do you think your child will feel about it?
6. Are you open to changing your mind about disclosure in the future? What factors do you think might make you change your mind?
7. Do you feel free to explore thoroughly the issues associated with third-party reproduction, both now and later? Why or why not?
8. What is the cost of the procedures you're considering?
9. What legal agreements are required?
10. What sort of medical screening does your clinic do on donors?
11. What sort of access do adult offspring have to donor records?
12. If you want a second child, would you want to use the same donor? Is this possible?
13. If the donor is a friend or relative, do you all agree on the degree of openness? What has been decided?
14. If you're considering embryo adoption, does the program you're considering have good success rates with thawed embryos?

Chapter 17

Using a Donor

What the Kids and the Research Tell Us

Often donor arrangements work beautifully. But they are not without some difficulty. For those who have prayerfully considered third-party reproduction and believe they have God's blessing on such a choice, we shift our focus to what some of the research tells us. Despite the many issues associated with donor eggs, donor sperm, and embryo adoption, many couples believe the benefits outweigh the problems.

The Benefits

The benefits of using a donor include the following:

1. Couples see some advantages when they compare using a donor to pursuing adoption. Many couples faced with third-party reproduction prefer it to adoption. One study showed that most couples had considered adoption before deciding instead to try donor insemination (DI). As with treatment for infertility, the adoption process is time-consuming, intrusive, and beyond the couple's control. Using a donor allows couples to avoid the "parent selection" process of adoption, in which they feel they must prove they are good enough to qualify as parents, and some couples may be ineligible for adoption (due to age or other factors). With DI, there's the additional advantage of expense. While adopting or in vitro fertilization (IVF) may cost more than $10,000, DI costs $1,500 or less, depending on a variety of factors, including whether the semen is shipped from overseas.

2. A child conceived through a DI has a decreased risk of known birth defects. Donors go through careful screening. If one of the spouses desiring children has a genetic disorder, using a donor virtually eliminates the worry about transmitting that particular disease.

3. The mother can control the baby's prenatal environment. Unlike an adoptive mom who wonders whether a birth mother used drugs or alcohol while carrying the child, the mother in a sperm-donor situation can decide exactly what will be ingested during pregnancy.

4. The mother can experience pregnancy, birth, and breastfeeding. For many infertile women, these are rites of womanhood.

5. One parent gets to contribute to the child's genetic makeup. While the infertile husband can't experience the joy of passing on his genes, his fertile wife can through DI. The reverse is true when a donor egg is used.

6. The child may be able to have a full genetic sibling. Some couples use the same donor more than once so their children are biological sisters and/or brothers.

7. The couple can keep their infertility private. Many couples would prefer to keep their infertility private, either because it's highly personal to them or because of a sense of shame over their inability to conceive. These couples see a donor as a chance to forget they are infertile and move on. Once the wife conceives, outsiders no longer assume the couple is infertile.

The Disadvantages

As a person conceived through DI, I believe it is essential to tell the child. First, I believe it should be the child's right to know the truth about his conception. Second, it's difficult to maintain such a vital secret for the lifetime of the child-adult relationship without a tangled web of deceptions. Third, the effects of keeping a secret will probably damage the child's ability to trust you. Fourth, most children are more perceptive than their parents think and will perceive that some kind of information is being withheld.[1]

Despite the advantages, there are some clear disadvantages to using a donor, some of which have become more apparent in recent years. These disadvantages are issues that couples must work through carefully before proceeding.

1. A donor arrangement has the potential to negatively impact the marriage relationship. One of the spouses is genetically connected to the child, while the other is not. It has been argued that though the "bypassed parent" has given consent, even if truly informed and uncoerced, that consent can hardly equalize the imbalance: "The intruding third-party donor, as in adultery, will inevitably be a psychological reality in the couple's life. Even if there is no jealousy or envy, the reproductive inadequacy of one partner has been ... superseded by an outsider's potency, genetic heritage, and superior reproductive capacity. Fertility and reproduction has been given an overriding priority in the couple's life."[2]

Some couples insist they do not have such an imbalance. But concern over the potential for this imbalance does raise questions about priorities and motives that the couple must at least explore. Is the infertile partner saying "Okay" because he or she is eclipsed by the other's negative feelings? Is she sensitive to how he feels about this and vice versa? Is he opting for DI, or is she opting for donor egg (DE), to hide something that makes them feel ashamed?

In a study of fifty-eight couples who had DI children, women had more positive experiences than men, with no measurable adverse effects. The women tended to be more willing than the men to inform the child about its DI origins. One of the concerns that surfaced in the study was whether DI had been chosen to build the father's social image as being masculine, though the arrival of the DI child did have a significant effect in improving his marital relationship. The data also showed that counseling prior to starting treatment brought about better outcomes.

Another study that included fifty DI couples found that they were poor assessors of how their partners felt. Females felt males were less happy than the men actually were; males perceived females as being more happy than the women actually were. The average husband's view of the donor was also more negative than that of his wife. Clearly, couples embarking on the donor-gamete journey need to have some heart-to-heart communication, perhaps aided by a counselor who is well acquainted with the issues.

2. DI and DE, unlike with adoption, involve the deliberate creation of a child. DI and DE have been likened to "half an adoption." Yet the donor offspring themselves have noted a key distinction: adoption of a child is an alternative solution to an unplanned, unintentional situation; donor conception is a deliberate creation of a child.

3. A religious and social stigma is often associated with third-party reproduction. In October 2002, the Israel Health Ministry granted permission to a couple to predetermine the gender of their child for religious reasons. The couple had asked for a daughter. Having opted for DI and wanting to keep the donor a secret, they realized they could do so only if the woman were to give birth to a female child. If they had a son, they would be able to keep the matter under wraps only until the boy turned thirteen. As the news story explained, "When the son of a

Cohen celebrates his bar mitzvah and goes up to read from the Torah, he is heralded in synagogue as a Cohen. In the case of the young couple, however, such an announcement would be a [violation], as the boy would not be the biological son of the father, and the parents would be forced to reveal the issue of the sperm donation.[3] To avoid this problem, the couple opted for a female embryo because a daughter would never go up to read from the Torah. Thus, their community wouldn't know that she was not their biological child, and they wouldn't have to tell her.

Often the stigma associated with DI drives couples to choose nondisclosure. Some insist that older generations (their parents, aunts, uncles, etc.) would not understand if they were to find out. Couples fear that the truth, were it known outside the nuclear family, would result in the child's mistreatment. If people say tacky things to infertile couples, they're going to say really inflammatory words to donor offspring. Parents want to avoid situations in which their children face others' judgments that make them feel different, insecure, and inferior, as though they must justify their origins. As one parent confided, "We need to protect children from the ignorant masses."

4. Donor offspring may need medical information about donors. Some DI offspring have discovered they were not genetically related to their fathers when they have run into situations where blood types didn't match or they needed organ donors and learned they didn't match their fathers or their siblings. Others have been diagnosed with genetic diseases and have desperately wanted information about their genetic histories.

As an adult adoptee who was not allowed medical information because my adoption records were closed, I'm angry and disappointed. More than 3,000 genetic diseases exist, and lives have been destroyed as adoptees have died due to secrecy, government barricades, and a system that polices people like criminals. [Supporting] anonymous donors of any kind is a sorry position. Sealing the identities of human beings as if they are in a witness protection program is like playing Russian roulette.

It is important to know one's original identity and one's medical and ancestral history. To deny a person his or her basic genetic information can have potentially serious negative consequences on that person's psychological, physical, and social well-being.

A mother of three donor offspring wrote: "Without information, many will have their health at risk unknowingly. Others will suffer with identity issues. Why should we cause injury to another when the answers are at hand?" An article in the *Ottawa Citizen* demonstrated this concern with the following:

> What Olivia Pratten knows about her biological father wouldn't fill a bubble gum baseball trading card. She has height, weight, eye and hair colour and blood type. The information is scribbled on a grubby, scrap piece of stationery a doctor handed her when she went looking for information about the stranger who helped create her.
>
> "Where's the health history?" Olivia demanded.
>
> "Don't worry, dear," the doctor told her. "I did a verbal check. The donor was healthy."
>
> Olivia stood on a Vancouver sidewalk two years ago staring down at that flimsy piece of paper. "This is it?" she thought. "This is all I have? This is crap."[4]

5. Donor offspring may accidentally marry close relatives. The risk of this happening is so minuscule as to make it almost not worth mentioning. Nevertheless, it's within the realm of possibility. The intended marriage partner would not be a full sibling but a half-brother or half-sister. The risk increases when a clinic does not greatly restrict the number of live births allowed per donor.

6. Parents who choose to keep information from their child about his or her identity violate the child's rights. Society is moving toward a culture of disclosure, in which children have the right to know their origins. This is such an important consideration that we will now explore it at length.

Scenarios—Open or Shut Case?

Couples face two key decisions when it comes to disclosure. The first is whether to insist on a donor who is willing to be identified. The second is whether to tell the child about the donor.

Identified Donor

In 2002, the British Broadcasting Corporation (BBC) asked eighty-two donors at three sperm banks how they would feel about allowing children to know their genetic fathers' identities. Fifty-three said that they would not continue to donate. In fact, if given the choice, approximately 70 percent of sperm donors elect to remain anonymous. Thus, clinics say they'll be unable to recruit donors if they have to reveal donors' identities. However, some donors *are* willing to enter open arrangements. In fact, it's often the parents, rather than donors, who are most insistent about maintaining anonymity. Today some U.S. clinics do offer identified donors. Some Swedish clinics have found that a shift in recruiting policies has resulted in an increased number of donors who were happy to be identified.

In the past, little identifying information was available, but today it is generally accepted that the more information available, the better. Couples wanting an anonymous donor need to explore their reasons. As they do so, we encourage them to consider these statements by donor offspring:

> *It's infuriating that most banks remain wedded to the idea that sperm donation has to be anonymous. They want to protect the donor as though he is a victim of some sort. But why should the medical profession have the power to deny someone his or her full genetic history?*

> *I'm curious to meet my genetic dad. I'm not looking for a father figure—I think of my dad as my real father. I just want information. I'd really like to ask him about himself.*

An adult adoptee commenting on DI had this to say: "I am not ungrateful for the sacrifices made by those who gave me life. Nor do I wish to 'trade in' the loving parents who raised me for the parents to whom I have genetic ties. I am simply trying to put together the puzzle that is my unique individuality."[5]

Not all those seeking their biological roots are as detached as the donor offspring quoted above. As with some adult adoptees who search for their biological parents, many donor offspring fantasize about an idealistic world in which loving donor parents will welcome them and forge meaningful connections. For these offspring, access to full genetic histories would be insufficient. More than justice is at stake, then. It goes beyond that to the level of need. Some clinics do provide an enormous amount of medical information without identifying features, but that does not stop the longing of some to meet the biological donor.

Most infertility clinics focus on helping infertile couples to have babies. But they are ill-equipped to support these couples as they think about the long-term implications of gamete donation.

Informed Child

The decision about whether to tell their child or children is the second major decision a couple must make when deciding whether to use a donor. Consider the differing choices the following two couples made.

Roy and Rebecca sought assistance with male-factor infertility after discovering Roy had no viable, motile sperm. As an only child himself and rather advanced in years, Roy wanted to proceed with DI, and his wife agreed. She conceived quickly. They decided early in the pregnancy to keep the procedure a complete secret from all parties, including the child. Their decision to keep this secret, even from their child, has remained firm.

Another couple, Tim and Carol, found after semenalysis that Tim had azoospermia (the complete absence of sperm in the seminal fluid). They elected donor insemination, and Carol was inseminated twice over a period of three years with the same donor, in both cases successfully. Their decision was revealed to family members and friends, who had been part of the support group through prayer and counsel. Tim had good support dealing with the circumstances, and the marriage was characterized by good communication. From the time their daughter could understand, they spoke openly with her about the donor. As she grew up, she couldn't remember a time when she didn't know about him. The family appeared stronger for the experience.

As Roy's and Rebecca's story illustrates, many couples elect not to tell donor-conceived children about their origins. For anyone considering donor gametes, the questions of whether to tell and who to tell are important. Couples who have decided against disclosure say, "If you make that choice, you must tell absolutely *no* one. A story, once told, tends to get broadcast like the nightly news. Once it's out, it can never be untold."

Some parents worry that informed children will reject them. The mother of a donor-conceived child asked, "Will he be happier and healthier day-to-day if he knows, and will there be more love? Probably not." Others agree with her, stressing that it puts too much burden on a child to carry such an emotional load. One writer emphasized: "Children would never understand why you have made the decisions you have made. And you shouldn't have to defend your decision."

Some people advise, "If you can't decide, consider not telling anyone for a time. You can take each day at a time and 'sleep on it' for a year or two, then decide when the time is right and the child is at an age when he or she can understand."

Everyone seems to agree that the child should learn the information only from his or her parents, not from someone else. Unlike Roy and Rebecca, Tim and Carol chose to tell even their friends. Some feel disclosure should extend only to the child, and when that child is mature enough, he or she gets to decide who else knows.

Parents do risk losing their child's trust if they choose nondisclosure but the information somehow comes out. One DI mom chose to inform her kids rather than take that chance. She described the time before she and her husband told their children as "living a lie." And a DI daughter describes what happened during her teen years when she learned about her conception during an argument between her parents: "I was very confused. But it was a relief that there wasn't something wrong with me." Some research indicates that many donor-conceived children whose parents opted not to tell them grew up with a sensation that something was being kept from them. Others, sensing something amiss at home, wondered, "Did Mom have an affair?"

Before the first wave of donor offspring was grown enough to have a voice on the topic, concern that the child might find out later and feel betrayed was considered the most important factor in the parents' decision in favor of disclosure. Sometimes the children *do* find out.

With the advent of greater information-sharing about adoption, more people now insist that the child's right to know is universal. As one expert put it: "There is now a strong current of thought that it is irresponsible to aid in the begetting not only of fatherless children but also of children who can never know who their fathers were." David Blankenhorn, author of the best-selling book *Fatherless America*, is strongly critical of what he calls "sperm fathers."[6] "Our essential identity is connected with our biological origins," according to Dr. John Fleming, director of the Southern Cross Bioethics Institute in Adelaide. "Rejecting the idea of fatherhood or seeing it as a tacked-on, optional extra is to deny the nature of human beings."[7] It is difficult to justify how it can be in the best interest of the child for him or her to be brought up in ignorance of half of his or her genetic inheritance.

Most social workers and counselors who work with donor offspring agree that disclosure between parent and child is the wisest course. Couples thinking of nondisclosure need to ask themselves how such a decision would fit with "Do unto others" (Luke 6:31) or biblical admonitions to practice the truth (1 John 1:6).

Studies have demonstrated that secrecy has several damaging effects. Families choosing to withhold the truth from their children potentially reinforce negative stereotypes about donors and ARTs, as well as violating social norms of interpersonal relations. One study of sixteen DI couples found that secrecy about DI hindered their ability to work through conflicts about infertility.

The same study revealed that one factor in the success of a DI arrangement was that those who waited for some time before forging ahead adjusted better to their infertility than those who didn't wait before pursuing DI. Other research demonstrates that those choosing disclosure have found that such openness has had little negative effect on the child or the family.

For those who conclude that third-party reproduction is allowable, considerations about disclosure require attention. Couples must explore both feelings about and motivations for using donor gametes before initiating donor arrangements. And they should consider the rights and needs of the potential children created from such arrangements.

In the past, donors' participation was contingent on anonymity. Now that more information is available about the effect of nondisclosure on donor offspring, we are not arguing about whether the rights and needs of adult offspring should nullify anonymity agreements. Our point is simply that while donor-recipient agreements were made in good faith, they were often made without data, or with little data, from the children's perspectives about the anonymity of their genetic parents. Now we have some data. We've included in this chapter what we now know from studies and interviews with DI offspring. (Most DE offspring are still too young to comment.) Thus, infertile couples facing decisions about third-party reproduction must make important decisions about disclosure, acting in the best interest of the child or children they long to create.

DISCUSSION QUESTIONS

1. If you are the fertile partner, how would you feel if you were the one unable to contribute your own gametes?
2. How would your family feel about your use of a donor?
3. What are the ramifications of such a choice in your religious community?
4. What is your theological and ethical understanding of third-party reproduction?
5. If you were to pursue counseling with a staff member at your clinic, would he or she respect your ethical construct?
6. What are your views on disclosure?

Chapter 18

LOSS UPON LOSS

MISCARRIAGE, FAILED IVF, AND FAILED ADOPTION

When sorrows come, they come not single spies, but in battalions ...
—William Shakespeare, *Hamlet*, act 4, scene 5

For my first pregnancy I was carefree. The following pregnancies were much different. After each subsequent loss, I focused more on the details of what I was doing, touching, having contact with, eating. At one point I refused to use deodorant because I was afraid of an ingredient that might cause miscarriage. I became the epitome of paranoia! Unfortunately, none of my efforts resulted in making any kind of difference.

I was unable to focus on my strengths, because I didn't feel I had any. I felt so lost, alone, and singled out for failure that I could hardly function. If it weren't for my pets, I probably wouldn't have gotten out of bed in the morning.

The inability to have children when you want them is devastating. Sadly, for a lot of couples, the infertility struggle gets even tougher as they experience additional losses in the process. Any loss of a long-awaited child can be hard—whether through miscarriage, ectopic pregnancy, failed adoption, the loss of one or more children in a multiple pregnancy,[1] a failed in vitro fertilization (IVF) cycle, or a stillbirth. But for the couple with years invested in trying to have a baby, the news is especially crushing. Infertility patients tend to experience these losses more intensely than those who get pregnant in the "regular world."

Miscarriage and Stillbirth

We had an early miscarriage, and I think some people think that it is not a big deal, but I was pregnant for a few short days. And in those days I bonded with my child and made all kinds of plans. My husband and I even looked on the internet for a crib together and looked up names. Just because we didn't have that joy for very long doesn't mean it still is not painful.

After our baby died, I read two Christian books. Afterward I felt worse—like if only I had enough faith, the pain would magically go away.

Fourteen years ago I gave birth to a baby girl. Four hours later she died. Doctors, nurses, and friends all said, "You're young. You'll have other babies. Try to forget."

A pregnancy loss that occurs before the twentieth week of gestation is officially called a "spontaneous abortion," more commonly known as "miscarriage." Loss after twenty weeks is called a "stillbirth."

Though couples who have experienced the trauma of such a loss sometimes wonder how so many people could have possibly survived it, pregnancy loss is actually a fairly common experience.

- Miscarriages happen in about 15 percent of ultrasound-confirmed pregnancies and in about 50 percent of all pregnancies.[2] Others put this figure even higher, suggesting that as many as three-quarters of all fertilized eggs are lost.[3]
- Assuming that a conservative one in four pregnancies end in miscarriage, there are close to one million pregnancy losses occurring every year in the United States alone.[4]
- Most pregnancy losses happen in the first twelve weeks.
- One in every 115 births is a stillbirth, meaning 2,600 American women have stillborn babies every year.[5]
- Many experiencing pregnancy loss are suffering the loss of at least their third consecutive pregnancy.

What causes pregnancy loss? The woman who loses a pregnancy typically finds herself constantly analyzing what she could have done differently. She chides herself with "I shouldn't have used that disinfectant," or "I shouldn't have gone camping," or "I should have listened when Grandma told me not to lift my arms above my head."

No compelling evidence links pregnancy loss with excessive work, reasonable exercise, sexual intimacy, previous use of birth control pills, stress, bad thoughts, nausea, vomiting, or even welding. The most common reason for pregnancy loss is chromosomal problems that happen randomly. In fact, studies tell us that in about 50 to 60 percent of early miscarriages, genetically abnormal embryos are the cause.[6] The most common embryonic defect is an abnormal number of chromosomes. The risk of miscarriage increases with the ages of both the father and the mother.

Hearing this, well-meaning friends often say, "Your loss was God's way of taking a child with serious birth defects." This is both cruel and unhelpful. It only raises more questions: "So why wouldn't God take this child before I even found out I was pregnant?"

While a single pregnancy loss is most likely the result of chromosomal abnormality in the fetus, repeated losses are thought to be triggered by maternal factors, including uterine structural imperfections, hormonal abnormalities, infection, autoimmune problems, and illness. Other factors contributing to pregnancy loss include environmental causes and blood incompatibility between the mother and the embryo. In most cases, the specific reason for the loss remains unidentified.

Nevertheless, it's difficult to convince a woman who has lost a pregnancy that she could not have *somehow* prevented this tragedy. Sometimes the husband, too, feels that he should have been able to "fix it"— to find a way to protect his wife and child from such trauma.

What are the types of early pregnancy loss? The earliest type of loss is a *biochemical pregnancy*, in which the pregnancy ceases to develop in the early weeks, before ultrasound evidence appears. We know that conception did occur because of the "pregnancy hormone" (HCG) detectable in the blood.

A so-called *blighted ovum* occurs when the placental portion of the embryo develops but the fetus does not. Using the term "blighted ovum" is both sexist and inaccurate, as it blames the female (ovum), when technically the egg is no longer an ovum once it is fertilized; it's a zygote, and whether or not it develops properly may be related to sperm, egg, or both. "Early miscarriage" is a more appropriate label.

The third type of early pregnancy loss is an *ectopic* or *tubal pregnancy*, in which the embryo implants in a fallopian tube or in a site outside of the uterus.

I left my job because returning to work became so difficult following the losses. Each time it got worse. It was difficult to schedule the infertility treatment appointments, and my managers would not work with me on the scheduling. Unemployment was the worst thing for my depression. I was even more isolated than before.

Mother's Day—such a difficult day. I struggled with feeling left out. Inside I felt like a mother because I had bonded with the babies I carried. It was hard to be the only person who acknowledged those babies. Yet being recognized on Mother's Day, when my children were not with me here on earth, was also a painful reminder of what I had lost. There is just no comfortable, painless way to get through that day.

As if one loss weren't enough, about 1 to 2 percent of women will have three or more miscarriages, which is called *recurrent pregnancy loss.* An underlying contributing factor can be identified 40 to 50 percent of the time. When a contributing factor is found and treated, the prognosis for successful pregnancy outcome is typically about 80 percent. Even when no underlying problem is found, the chances for a successful pregnancy can typically be in the 50 to 70 percent range.[7] Almost anyone who has lost a pregnancy worries about subsequent losses, and in the past, many doctors waited until the third miscarriage to begin testing for underlying problems. More recent information suggests testing should take place after two losses, especially for women over thirty. Newer studies indicate a miscarriage rate of 26 to 40 percent after a woman has suffered two losses, so earlier testing makes sense emotionally, physically, and in many cases, financially as well.[8]

Why do we feel so terrible about the loss of a pregnancy?

Sometimes I feel afraid I'm taking too long to overcome grief, but then I try to remember everyone has a different timing, and that my grandma's eyes still shine with a tear when she talks about a baby girl she lost forty-five years ago.

My husband and I suffered a loss at eleven weeks, so we never planned a memorial service. We did attend a healing mass for parents who have suffered child loss. We have also planted a tree in our yard in honor of our baby. These things were helpful in our healing process. When we get ready for bed, we always say a quiet prayer for all the members of our families and then we hold hands and ask God to watch over us and protect us. We also give each other an extra kiss for our baby.

Depending on one's personality and background, each person's response to the loss of a pregnancy varies. Men and women generally have different feelings about these losses as well, with women tending to feel more of a bond with the child that was lost. And sadly, many comforters overlook the husbands when expressing compassion. Flowers and cards get sent to the mother, and people who bring meals walk right past the men without stopping to offer solace. Friends tend to direct all their words and expressions of touch to the young mother who has just suffered the loss. And because many husbands grieve more privately than their wives, the wives may have an increased sense that they are suffering alone.

While infertility is an expanded, drawn-out loss, miscarriage is a compressed loss. Yet the emotions and perceptions are often the same—only magnified with miscarriage. And the intensity of that pain depends on a number of factors, the most significant of which is the couple's psychological investment in the pregnancy. Often the longer couples have been trying to conceive, the greater their sense of loss. Also, though 75 percent of pregnancy losses occur before the end of the twelfth week, they can occur at any time during the forty-week gestation period. Some couples experience added grief because they believed the misconception that "once you get past the third month, you're home free."

According to one psychologist, the wave of grief often crests and begins to subside between three and nine months after the loss, although some report that it takes between eighteen months and two years. And the healing process can be disrupted by other life difficulties, including further fertility treatment.

Pregnancy Loss as a Spiritual Journey: Maureen and Erik's Story

Maureen: "After trying for two years, I finally got pregnant. We were ecstatic. We didn't know if we should tell anyone, so we waited more than a month before informing our parents. Around eight weeks' gestation, I started having spotting. I went in for an ultrasound, and we were overjoyed to see a heartbeat. A few weeks later, I had some cramping, so I went alone to see the doctor because my husband was in a meeting. When the doctor did the ultrasound, we found no heartbeat. Erik passed me on the way home, and he immediately knew by the look on my face what had happened. After that, I didn't leave the house for two weeks. I was a mess—a total mess.

"Erik dumped his schedule, and we stayed home. I couldn't sleep at night. I napped a lot during the day and watched movies and Christmas shows. I was trying to avoid having a D&C, but when my husband found me crawling in pain, he took me to the hospital in a wheelchair.

"They put me in the maternity ward ... with all the baby pictures. I got the crummiest room they had—it was the size of a closet. I walked around saying, 'I can't believe we're here.'"

Erik: "My best man from our wedding came to the hospital and stayed until 3 A.M. We watched TV and talked. It was nice to have someone around.

"For two weeks my wife and I just held each other and cried and didn't talk about it. Then after two weeks, we went out to Starbucks, and we sat and asked the hard questions. What does it mean from God? What happens to infants when they die?

"Someone had told me that God must have meant that to be. I was mad. Through the whole thing, I've sensed God's peace, even through extreme pain. The world is broken; it's not as it's supposed to be, but Jesus is redeeming people. And someday we won't have all this [brokenness]. In a weird way, that's comforting. A few people have quoted Romans 8:28 about how all things work together for good. We smile and inside say, 'Just shut up.' Sometimes I put on a nice Christian face and mentally swear at them. Truth be told, at one point I literally flipped God off. Then I thought, 'That was a stupid thing to do.' So I repented. But I also demanded, 'Where were you?' But then I realized, 'You were there all along. Why did it happen? I don't know, but I still trust You.' How do you survive this without knowing who God is?"

Ectopic Pregnancy

Several years after we adopted our daughter, Alexandra, I (Sandi) conceived spontaneously. But on the day I was supposed to have the ultrasound, I started experiencing sharp abdominal pain, shortness of breath, and a racing pulse.

Uh-oh . . .

The doctor took a look via sonography that afternoon. Nothing showed up in the uterus. We stared at the screen as he moved the trans-vaginal probe to take a look at the tube. Then he asked us a rather odd question: "What are your plans for the evening?"

"Emergency surgery, right?"

He sighed. "I'm afraid so." He shook his head. "I'm sorry."

The pregnancy was in the fallopian tube.

In the case of an ectopic (or tubal) pregnancy, the embryo implants in a fallopian tube or an extrauterine site, necessitating removal of the pregnancy before the tube ruptures, if possible. An alternative approach is to use a chemotherapy agent, methotrexate, to destroy the growing pregnancy in an effort to avoid surgery. This has proven successful in early ectopic pregnancies. Yet the thought of taking a poison to "cure" an abnormal pregnancy can be quite traumatic. At this point we have *no* way to save the pregnancy or move the pregnancy to a more desirable location. So the medical team, pastoral care team, and the patient and her spouse must focus on saving her life and trying to preserve her fertility.

An ectopic pregnancy can be life-threatening to the mother and is virtually always fatal to the child. Only on that *extremely* rare occasion when implantation occurs on the intestines or other abdominal structures, having extruded itself from the tube, can a baby occasionally survive to viability. But this is very risky to the mother. Should the pregnancy implant in the interstitial area (the part of the tube that passes through the uterine wall), so that the embryo is *almost* but not quite there, the risk of serious maternal hemorrhage is high, owing to the proximity of small arteries. The risk of maternal hemorrhage is also significant if the pregnancy implants in the cervix. The doctor determines precisely where the pregnancy implanted by using quality ultrasound. Once the location is known, the physician can then determine whether treatment by surgery (laparoscopy) or medication (methotrexate) would be best.

In about one in 6,000 pregnancies, a so-called heterotopic gestation occurs, in which one embryo implants inside the uterus and another implants in the tube or elsewhere. This may be as high as one in 100 following IVF and embryo transfer.[9]

Unfortunately, it's currently impossible to take an embryo from the tube and reimplant it in the uterus. Well-meaning people who suggest prayer and waiting upon God to "see if the pregnancy will 'migrate'" are dangerously misguided. This is equivalent to telling someone with crushing chest pain to pray and wait for the pain to move. If cholesterol plaques clog your arteries and trigger a heart attack, you hope that someone will rush you to the emergency room. Ectopic pregnancy is just as dangerous to a mother's life, and *close* medical observation is required, as ectopic pregnancy is currently the number one cause of maternal death in America for women in the first trimester of pregnancy.

The main risk factors for ectopic pregnancy, according to a large population-based study, are a history of sexually transmitted diseases and current smoking. The study looked at 803 women who had experienced ectopic pregnancy, and it found that women smoking more than twenty cigarettes a day were four times more likely to have an ectopic pregnancy than nonsmokers. Women with a history of pelvic inflammatory disease had more than triple the risk of ectopic pregnancy compared to the population at large.[10] Other risk factors include a history of infertility, age, previous miscarriages, previous IUD use, previous pelvic or abdominal surgery, and endometriosis. In addition, the risk of an etopic pregnancy is nearly three times greater if a woman has had a medically induced abortion (using RU-486). No increased risk has been noted after surgical abortion.[11]

Symptoms of ectopic pregnancy include vaginal bleeding, shoulder pain (referred pain from irritation of the diaphragm due to the blood in the abdomen), and some weakness or dizziness caused by blood loss and lowered blood pressure. A patient with an ectopic pregnancy will often get dizzy or pass out when standing up.

Sometimes methotrexate (taken orally or as a shot in the hip) doesn't work; the HCG level continues to climb or holds steady instead of falling. When this is the case, the patient will need surgery.

There are some rare pregnancy disorders following ectopic pregnancies or miscarriages. These disorders involve a cancer-like transformation of the placental tissue. HCG levels must be monitored to confirm that this rare situation is not present and that physical healing is complete.

Cases in which the pregnancy is too far along to be treated with medication require surgery. Sometimes it will be impossible to save the involved tube; in rarer cases, the uterus will be lost as well. If the tubes are undamaged, chances of conceiving again are good. Even if a damaged tube must be removed, many women conceive with only one tube. However, once a woman has suffered one ectopic pregnancy, the chances of recurrence are higher.

I have experienced two ectopic pregnancies. Both were treated with a "wait and see" approach and methotrexate. This was especially hard on my husband and me because of the added danger of losing my life and/or fertility.

The only emotion my husband displayed was the relief that I was going to be okay. He has told me several times that he thought I was going to die. He was extremely worried about me—even more than he was worried about us losing the baby. He feels so blessed to still have me.

An ectopic pregnancy can bring a bundle of mixed emotions in addition to the usual grief caused by pregnancy loss. Relief that the wife's life has been spared is mixed with sadness over losing the child. In addition, anytime a woman experiences pregnancy loss of any kind, her body goes through enormous upheaval, with physical and emotional ramifications that arise in part because of the incredible hormonal shifts associated with pregnancy. It may take up to six weeks or even longer for a woman to feel like herself again physically, and the normal grieving process takes much longer.

Failed IVF Cycle

We were at the threshold of those frightening words: IVF. Then I thought, "It will have to work. There is no real reason for it not to, even at the first try. If not this, then what? There was no "I could handle a failure." It just could not, would not, happen. When it failed, you can imagine our sorrow and shock.

That was the hardest call, when the doc phoned to say the test was negative after IVF. It hit me so hard that I couldn't get myself to say anything but "Why? What happened?" His answer: "I wish something would have gone wrong. Maybe then I would have known why."

Michelle, a chaplain, was discussing how she could set up a support network for couples who had experienced pregnancy loss. When it was suggested that she might want to also include couples who had gone through failed IVF cycles, her eyes suddenly welled with tears. Then her own story began to unfold.

She and her husband had been through treatment with no success. Finally their reproductive endocrinologist recommended IVF. When the time came, several eggs were fertilized and transferred. It was hard for her not to get carried away by the feeling of being pregnant—knowing those embryos were alive at transfer.

But then the bad news. After only a few weeks, the spotting began. A blood test confirmed her fears; she was not pregnant. Michelle was both shocked that the embryos had died and astounded at the intensity of her own grief.

Several months passed, and still no relief came. The failed IVF cycle represented both the deaths of her children and the death of any hope of conceiving. For Michele, it was the end of the road. Part of her grief, she said, was over a sense of not belonging in any clear category. She didn't feel she could seek solace in a miscarriage support group. The grief was like phantom pains.

Some have wondered if IVF has a higher than average miscarriage rate. Actually, the miscarriage rate among women who undergo ART procedures is on par with that of women who conceive naturally. A team evaluated the miscarriage rate among more than 60,000 pregnancies stemming from ART procedures done in U.S. clinics between 1996 and 1998 and found the following:

- The miscarriage rate among ART pregnancies was 14.7 percent—similar to rates among pregnancies reported in the National Survey of Family Growth.
- Among nondonor, fresh-embryo pregnancies, the miscarriage rate ranged from 10.1 percent among women in their twenties to 39 percent among women older than forty-three.
- Women who used donor eggs had a miscarriage rate of 13.1 percent, with little variation among different age groups.

- Overall, the miscarriage rate *was* somewhat higher among women whose pregnancies were conceived with frozen and thawed embryos compared with those who received freshly fertilized embryos.
- Pregnancies in which the mother was carrying only one child had a higher miscarriage rate than those in which she carried twins, triplets, or more.[12]

If you have experienced a loss following an IVF cycle—whether your embryos didn't survive, you had a miscarriage, or you lost one or more children in a multiple gestation—grief is a normal response to your situation. Couples who experience such losses have nothing tangible to connect them to their child—no lock of hair, no photograph—so they often struggle with the pain they feel, even doubting whether the pain is legitimate. It certainly is. That tiny life is of infinite, eternal worth to the Creator. A human life has been lost, and grief over that loss is real and valid.

If you have experienced a failed IVF cycle in which no fertilization occurred, you too have been through enormous emotional and physical upheaval. You need time, empathy, patience, compassion, kindness, and encouragement to talk without having to hear solutions. You are not alone!

Failed Adoption

Shelley called to say she had changed her mind about giving us her baby. Her pastor advised her that, having made the decision that led to getting pregnant, she needed to take full responsibility for the consequences by raising the baby herself.

Couples who are expecting a child through adoption suffer emotionally when the birth parents change their minds. Having formed emotional ties with the birth mother (and sometimes with the birth father) and particularly with the expected child, the couple once again experiences the loss of dreams. If the adoptive parents have already taken physical custody, the trauma is even greater.

If you have experienced this kind of loss, perhaps you will identify with the expressions of sadness and hope made by others who have been through similar experiences.

I feel so old; I wanted to have a baby before I was thirty-five.

For so long, people have said, "You can always adopt." Now that our adoption has fallen through, I wonder if we will ever be able to have any children.

For the first time I'm really struggling with anger at God. I'm learning that it's okay to feel whatever I feel, but I have to remember that it's within the context of a relationship. We may say, "It's okay to get mad at God," but we also need to say, "Now it's time to apologize," like we would in any other relationship.

I do a shabby job of being gracious. It's pretty hard to cut people slack when you're at the edge of yourself.

In prayer I'm feeling more convinced that the only things we can confidently believe God to do are the things he has revealed he will do . . . give wisdom, peace, grace.

No matter which of these losses is experienced, men and women find they are unprepared for the anguish that follows. It may take a long time to heal from the emotional trauma of such a loss. And as with other aspects of infertility, men and women typically handle their grief differently. The wife tends to feel more incapacitated; her husband often feels he must carry on. Sometimes his seeming ability to function normally makes her wonder if he ever cared in the first place.

Often the kinds of losses discussed in this chapter are not discussed in public, so most people don't realize how debilitating the grief can be. And while many people may sympathize—however imperfectly—with the couple that has lost a pregnancy through stillbirth, miscarriage, or ectopic pregnancy, few recognize the pain of a failed IVF attempt, the loss of one child in a multiple pregnancy, or a failed adoption, whether or not the child was already placed in the couple's home. Yet these losses of children and dreams can be excruciating, and a heightened sensitivity is in order. If you have experienced such a loss, allow yourself time to express and work through your anguish, knowing that your grief is a healthy expression of mourning what could have been.

DISCUSSION QUESTIONS

1. Have you experienced any of the losses described? If so, what was your experience? Your spouse's experience?
2. If you've been through such a loss, did you feel polarized from your spouse? If so, how did you work through it? Are you allowing yourself to acknowledge that a human life has been lost?
3. Do you need a break from treatment to allow extra time for working through the pain? If so, how long do you think you need?
4. Do you know anyone who has experienced any of these types of losses? How did they respond?
5. Have you encountered those who believe ectopic pregnancy can "migrate to the uterus"? If so, what did you say? How would you respond if you were to encounter such a person?
6. What, if any, misconceptions have you heard about stillbirth, miscarriage, failed IVF cycles, and/or failed adoption?
7. Did you identify with any of the stories or quotes presented in this chapter? Why or why not?
8. If you have experienced one or more of the losses described in this chapter, how would you say you are coping? What stage are you at in processing your grief? Would you describe yourself right now as being primarily in a stage of denial, anger, depression, mourning, or resolution?
9. Might a tangible acknowledgment of your loss, such as planting a tree or holding a memorial service help? (The *Book of Common Prayer* includes prayers for those who have lost children in its service of Burial for the Dead.)

Chapter 19

INFERTILITY PATIENT AS PARENT

SECONDARY INFERTILITY, PREGNANCY, AND PARENTING AFTER INFERTILITY

Secondary Infertility

Caught between two worlds—fertile and infertile. And excluded from both!

Arranging childcare can be difficult, and babysitting gets expensive. Going to an infertility clinic can be stressful. A child in a waiting room full of infertile women—there's the stare factor.

Can you pay for infertility treatments and still save for your child's education?

Primary infertility patients—those with no children—hear "just relax" and "just adopt." Secondary infertility patients—those who have one or more children but have been unable to have another—hear their own set of insensitive remarks. Sadly, some of these remarks come from primary infertility patients:

- At least you have one child. You should be grateful.
- Stop worrying. Your body has proved it can do it. It'll happen; it just takes time.
- He's an only child? Don't you want to give him a brother or a sister? He'll be so spoiled.

The American Society for Reproductive Medicine (ASRM) estimates that 1.3 million women in the United States suffer from secondary infertility. Others place that number as high as 3 million.[1] These couples, most of whom conceived easily when they started their families, suddenly realize it is not going to be easy to get pregnant again. Infertility after the birth of a first child is more common now than it was even in the mid-1990s, due in part to a growing trend toward delayed marriage and childbearing. Women with secondary infertility are about 40 percent *less* likely to seek medical assistance than are women with primary infertility.[2]

The causes of secondary infertility are often the same as for primary infertility, including irregular ovulation, endometriosis, and uterine fibroids. Infection also plays a major role. In addition, some secondary infertility cases stem from trauma received during a first pregnancy or delivery.

When Charla and Bob tried to have a second child, they were shocked to discover they had a fertility problem. It had been so easy the first time; it never occurred to them that they might have difficulty the second time. Having repeatedly told themselves, "But it worked once already," they waited a long time before seeking treatment.

Psychologists confirm that both primary and secondary infertility evoke feelings of guilt, denial, anger, depression, and frustration. But differences exist. Couples with secondary infertility often feel they fall between fertility and infertility. The fertile population generally perceives them as having no problem because they have a child. As a result, when in the company of primary infertility patients, secondary infertility patients often feel too ashamed to ask for support, for fear of evoking resentment. And they endure questions from the fertile population about when they plan to have another child (this also happens to couples who have adopted). Couples with secondary infertility must function as parents as they grieve their absent child or children.

Debra, who returned to fertility treatment after having a high-tech baby, says the second time through treatment she felt a different kind of pain: "Now that I have one child I've exchanged the anguish of having no children for the pain of knowing exactly what I'm missing the second time." Another mom finds that an activity as common as picking up her daughter from kindergarten brings unexpected grief: "You notice you're the only mother who is not pregnant, carrying an infant, or holding a toddler's hand. Your child asks why she's the only one in her class who has no brothers or sisters. You listen to everyone in your play group discuss how far apart they want to space their children, and then you watch them conceive according to plan. You press on with temperature charts, medications, and doctor visits. You wonder if your child will be emotionally scarred by your deep desire to have another child. You struggle to answer friends and relatives who comment, 'Time for another, isn't it?' Or worse, you search for an answer to those who say, 'You have one child. Be grateful.'"

Patients with secondary infertility also face other difficult situations. There's the question about what to do with maternity clothes. And if it's painful to serve in the church nursery, couples feel guilty opting out of the rotation assigned to all parents of young children. It may be hard, too, for secondary infertility patients to know what to tell their child. One patient says, "My daughter ends her prayers nightly with, 'Please give us a baby.'"

"It's nearly impossible to explain to someone who feels their family is complete why you grieve for the phantom child," says Charla. "People try to tell us we should feel satisfied with the child we have. I compare it to how I feel about my mother. She died a few months before my daughter was born. I feel grateful to God for giving me a wonderful mother, but no matter how grateful I feel, it never takes away my longing to be with her. Gratitude never replaces longing."

Another patient agrees. "I'm grateful that I have this child. The fact that I grieve doesn't take away from my gratefulness. But there's still an empty place in my heart."

Secondary infertility often brings guilt in a variety of forms. Many moms and dads chide themselves about the quality of their parenting. They often wonder if some curse has been cast on them for being terrible parents the first time. When their child misbehaves—as all children do—the parents may tell themselves, "No wonder we're not supposed to have another."

Many couples find that secondary infertility also complicates the adoption question. They worry about real or perceived equality in homes with a biological-adoptive mix. Some agencies turn away couples with a biological child. Also, many agencies have a ceiling on parental age. And because secondary infertility affects couples with at least one child, they are typically older than childless infertility patients.

Along with the worry and guilt comes fear. Many patients fear their child will be lonely, lacking family connections. The parents may become overly protective or unusually ambitious for their one child. They're concerned that their child will be spoiled. And they fear that their only child will die, leaving them with no legacy. They also fret about the future of the child, envisioning one person bearing alone the burden of aging parents.

U.S. Census Bureau statistics indicate that close to 20 percent of all families have only one child. Further research indicates that this number will increase to 25 percent in the near future. The average family size in the United States is decreasing, and in fact, over the past few decades, the percentage of one-child families has increased faster than any other family type, so that today more than 15.5 million American families have only one child.

One advantage to having only one child is that it's becoming more socially acceptable. Far from being self-centered brats, only children score quite high on sociability indexes, meaning that in terms of relationships with their peers, they are doing better than just fine. And they score even higher than firstborns in leadership ability and maturity. They also do well on tests of intelligence, achievement, and self-esteem.[3]

Many of the same feelings and situations that secondary infertility patients face are also experienced by couples who have adopted a child and must decide whether to do so again.

"Couples confronting secondary infertility need empathy and validation of their pain," says therapist Judy Calica. "They need the freedom to grieve their losses and they need support in resolving their crisis." And crisis it is. One secondary infertility patient, Stacia, describes the emptiness she feels over being unable to conceive again, saying, "This is the *most* difficult thing I've ever dealt with. I know I will always feel like I'm just not finished."

Pregnancy after Infertility

While secondary infertility is a unique struggle deserving special empathy, another group that gets far too little support is couples who conceive after experiencing infertility, which is more than half of all infertility patients.

Now that I'm eight months pregnant, I've been thinking about how having a baby doesn't erase infertility. You'd think it would, but all those years of monthly disappointments, treatments, and knowing that it takes a miracle plus huge medical intervention to get pregnant have changed who I am. Infertility is a part of me. Seems strange. I still hate Mother's Day. I suspect I always will.

I used to kind of resent it when patients who were pregnant after infertility continued coming to our support group. But now I totally understand why they did.

I dreamed of that moment—how I would scream with excitement when the doctor told me I was finally pregnant. But when that moment came, all I could do was ask, "Are you sure?" I felt that familiar surge of self-protection. "What if I lose the pregnancy?" I thought pregnancy would be the end, but it's only the beginning. It's terrifying!

It seems unfair that I don't feel the freedom to say, "We're going to have a baby!" Instead I say, "We're expecting." I'm not sure we'll actually

*have a baby. Infertility robbed me of that carefree joy. I've been through
too much to think it'll all work out great.*

Making the Announcement

A patient feels a swirl of mixed emotions, both positive and negative, when her infertility buddies announce their pregnancies. The infertile friend hearing the news of yet another pregnancy can feel
abandoned by a fellow "club member." When Susan finally conceived
after sharing the mutual bond of infertility with a coworker, she knew
her good news would both delight and hurt her friend. Finally she sent
a note that said, "I've written this to you three times. I keep tearing it up
because it's too hard to say. The fact is, infertility is just plain hard. I
want you to know I had a positive pregnancy test this week. Call me
when you feel like it. Believe me, I'll understand."

Rabbi Michael Gold, author of *And Hannah Wept*, says, "A couple
having a baby must share their good news with infertile friends in as
sensitive a way as possible. I will always remember a beautiful phone
call from a woman in my synagogue who had just given birth to a
healthy baby boy. She told me that although she and her husband were
overjoyed, they kept thinking of us. They knew that calls like theirs had
to be hard for us, but they were praying that we would be blessed with
a child soon. Her words brought tears to my eyes."

Sometimes, despite the fact that they've hated pregnancy announce-
ments for so long, infertile couples who finally conceive expect their
infertile friends to be overjoyed for them. After all, their infertile friends
know exactly what the couple has been through up to that point! Yet
expecting these friends to rejoice—at least initially—may be asking too
much. Not only may the news be a grief trigger, but it may also evoke
a sense of abandonment. So no matter how much a pregnant patient
wants her infertility buddies to scream and hug her when she has good
news, she still needs to consider writing notes to these friends. That
allows them to endure the initial shock in private and then to offer con-
gratulations when they're ready.

"I'm glad she got out. I ran to call and congratulate her," says a
patient whose fellow sufferer sent her a note saying she'd finally conceived. Still, she acknowledges, receiving the note was easier than having to handle that moment of realization face-to-face.

Both sides need to show compassion and maturity, thinking of others' needs before their own. The patient who has dreamed of a huge celebration when she has good news may have to lay to rest yet another
dream destroyed by infertility. And her infertile friends should avoid

minimizing her feelings—the very action they so often detest in members of the fertile population.

Even Good News Has Its Challenges

Fertility patients often imagine hearing "You're pregnant," believing it will be the end of their troubles. Yet even that news, joyous as it is, brings its own set of problems.

I asked the nurse a question and she started talking about the placenta. I had to ask her to back up and tell me what the placenta was. I could rattle off FSH [follicle-stimulating hormone] levels, follicle cm sizes, and the right uterine lining measurements for maximum potential, but I didn't know what a placenta was. I'd never let myself read that far.

With a high-risk pregnancy, I'm on complete bed rest. The isolation at home is very upsetting.

When I started having back problems and preterm labor, I felt I had to be stoic and take it all with a smile, grateful that I'd made it this far. I didn't feel I could share any of this with my infertile friends, the people who had been my emotional lifeline.

Pregnant patients tend to identify far more with members of the infertile, rather than the fertile, population. But infertile friends consider pregnant patients as "graduates" from the group, sometimes even ostracizing them as "the lucky ones."

Another transition that's usually tougher than the pregnant patient imagined is the change from fertility patient to obstetrics patient. She's been on a first-name basis with the staff, she's shown up a couple of times a week at midcycle, and she knows the inner workings of the medical office. She's also used to having sonograms several times a month. Now she's pregnant. She gets referred to an ob-gyn, and suddenly she feels like it's "take a number." There's often no strong sense of urgency when she calls with concerns. Nobody knows her by name. And the doctors are reluctant to do sonograms without a pressing medical reason.

In addition, a difficult pregnancy often lies ahead for the former infertility patient. Yet she has sworn, "If I ever get pregnant, I'll never complain!" As a result, her infertility continues to rob her of something—in this case, of the support she might receive during a tough pregnancy. Any whimpering is met with, "You asked for this!" if not verbally from others, in her own accusing self-talk. If she miscarried in the past, she's terrified throughout the pregnancy, especially until she makes it past the point at which she lost the previous baby. No one in the doctor's office comprehends why every twinge and pain requires—no, demands—immediate attention.

Couples who conceive after infertility, particularly those who conceive after in vitro fertilization (IVF), differ from those who conceive by natural means. They need additional support. The women tend to have more muscle tension and anxiety about losing the pregnancy; the men often have more indirect aggression, guilt, and detachment. The men also tend to be more anxious about losing the pregnancy and about the baby being abnormal.[4]

"I was thrilled to be pregnant after infertility," wrote one patient. "But it still had its challenges. Were they worth it? Of course. But it wasn't the end of the journey by any means. It was just a path to a beautiful destination that still had some rocks and fallen trees obstructing the road in places."

Parenting after Infertility: "I Asked for It, Right?"

When you have prayed and cried, and prayed and begged for eight agonizing years that God would fulfill your desire for children, it is hard simply to switch gears. I've become so accustomed to guarding my heart against disappointment, not letting myself anticipate too much, never letting too much hope spring up in my heart.

It took me a while to feel a bond with other parents of multiples, as I didn't feel I could request the help I needed when the kids were infants. I'd "asked" for this challenge, and I guess I thought I should be able to figure out how my husband and I could cope with it ourselves.

Those who parent after infertility—whether they build their families through birth or adoption—face a unique set of difficulties. One is getting beyond "forever grateful" mode so they can be normal parents. That's not to suggest they should be ungrateful! But vowing never to complain about children is as unrealistic as a single woman vowing never to think a negative thought about her husband, if only she could find one. Perhaps you've made such a vow:

- If I had a child, I'd be thankful for every hour of lost sleep I missed!
- If I had a child, I'd never complain.
- If I had a child, I'd never get irritated when she acted up in the grocery store.

Even if you haven't made such statements, perhaps your friends treat you as if you have. When your child vomits on you as you're on your way to an important meeting, you don't need to hear, "Hey, I warned you! You prayed for this! This is what you wanted." (Don't be surprised by such comments; if infertility teaches anything, it's that people will be insensitive.) Such words serve as reminders that infertility makes you different forever.

It's time to let the past go. Marriage means two self-centered sinners uniting together; having children means adding a tiny, self-centered critter (or more) to the mix. Of course you're going to be frustrated sometimes! Apart from grace and the empowerment of the Holy Spirit, marriage and family life will never reach the levels of intimacy God intended.

People in the fertile population sometimes assume infertile couples want kids so much only because they've idealized parenting, but most infertility patients realize parents have days when children bring frustration and even heartache. To infertility patients, that risk is better than having no children at all, as Betsy discovered.

After working with her local doctor for several years, Betsy's options for seeking more specialized infertility care were limited. Seeing the nearest specialist would have required long treks to the city, so when Danocrine therapy failed to cure her condition, she and her husband, Mark, applied for an adoption.

Betsy was unsentimental about the biological processes involved in motherhood. In fact, she had said, "One advantage of adoption is that you don't have to hassle with nursing or suffer the pain of childbirth."

"What about the 'part of being a woman' stuff?" a friend asked.

"Naaah. For me, I just want a baby."

Shortly after Thanksgiving, Betsy and Mark jangled their families out of their slumbers with phone calls to announce baby Devin's arrival through adoption. Frequent updates from the new parents followed. This child fulfilled their dreams of a happy, blue-eyed, round-faced Gerber baby.

Then one evening several months after Devin joined her family, Betsy's usually chipper voice at the other end of the receiver betrayed to a friend that Betsy was upset.

"What happened?"

"I just had to talk to you!" Betsy sobbed as she blurted out the words. "But it's so dumb . . . I feel awful even admitting it." Her crying slowed down to sniffles. "I've been grieving all day about my infertility. I really love my daughter, so I feel guilty even feeling this way."

"Did something trigger your feelings?"

"Yeah. My friend Mary Kay was at Mother's Day Out. She just had her fourth child, so we talked about our new babies. She invited me to see their videotape of the birth, assuring me it was 'tastefully filmed.' So we went to her place. I honestly thought I'd enjoy it." Betsy paused and sighed. "I was unprepared for what I saw. There was *my* doctor delivering *her* baby. The way he rejoiced in that delivery made it so special for Mary Kay and Jim. Then there were the touching moments between husband and wife. I was devastated that we'd missed out on all that. So I started crying. Mary Kay felt terrible, which made me feel worse. I assured her it wasn't her fault, and then I drove home. I've been crying all afternoon. I feel like we did all the work and somebody else got the party. My doctor and his staff labored with us, and the two of us spent a lot of money and emotional energy. Yet all of us as a team never had an event that provided closure. So I guess it does hurt that I'll never give birth. Childbirth feels like more than part of being woman; it's also part of being a wife. And after infertility, it's even part of being a patient."

She sighed deeply. "I thought we'd put infertility behind us. I adore our daughter. Yet there are scars I don't even know about that can reopen anytime. Tell me it's okay to grieve when they do—that it's okay to weep once in a while, even after the happy ending."

Those who have wondered, "Will the pain ever go away?" find, through years of parenting, that the pain does get mostly erased through time. Barbara Eck Menning, founder of RESOLVE, described her lingering lifetime grief as being like "an old friend" that showed up periodically. But it can be bittersweet rather than bitter. With each milestone, parents can remind themselves, "I thought I'd never have a child in the school play; I thought I'd never have a kid to take Christmas caroling; I thought we'd never sing Happy Birthday to our own child ... and here we are!"

Still, many infertility patients who adopt do experience a phenomenon similar to postpartum depression.[5] And for that minority of patients who have viewed the arrival of a child or children as the end of all suffering, the pain of reality can be crushing. Some families find that the stress of infertility and adoption have so strained their relationships that they never quite recover, even after the happy news. (Biological parents sometimes experience this same process of expectation and disappointment.) So infertile couples are wise to guard themselves from thinking the pregnancy or adoption will usher in utopia.

Those who anticipate parenting with realistic expectations ultimately approach it more creatively. And whereas biological parents look for those traits they are passing down—"Maybe she will be an artist like you or an engineer like me"—adoptive parents gaze in wonder at the blossoming personality before them, studying it so they can guide it into whatever it wants to be.

Other benefits can emerge from the pain, too. Researchers at London's Clinical and Health Psychology Research Centre at City University studied 184 families—43 with a naturally conceived child, 41 with an IVF child, 45 with a DI (donor insemination) child, and 55 with an adopted child—looking at the quality of parenting in each group. Results showed that mothers of adopted, DI, and IVF children expressed greater warmth and had a deeper level of emotional involvement with their child than did mothers with a naturally conceived child. And both mothers and fathers in these three groups showed greater interaction with their child than did parents who conceived naturally. The infertile parents also scored better on the stress test.[6]

While those who end up parenting must guard themselves lest they spoil and overprotect the child that took seven years, three IVFs, and $100,000 to conceive, those years of longing and loss can add to, rather than take away from, the preciousness of the long-awaited gift. One father who had experienced infertility as a young man still teared up at age seventy when describing the joy of holding his baby girl for the first time. An onlooker noted, "How often do you see dads getting that emotional fifty years after a normal delivery?"

DISCUSSION QUESTIONS

1. Do you feel that those who desire another child are ungrateful for what they have?
2. How have you perceived and responded to secondary infertility patients?
3. What do you think when people express how hard it is to be a parent?
4. How have you responded when your infertile friends have conceived?
5. If you are part of an infertility support group, are pregnant patients allowed to attend? Why or why not?
6. How do you want to be told when a fellow member of your infertility network conceives?
7. Have you made any unrealistic promises such as, "If I ever have a child, I'll never complain about sleepless nights," that might keep you from getting needed support in the future?
8. How can you and your spouse comfort each other when you find out another friend is pregnant? How would you like each other to respond?

Chapter 20

RESOLUTION

ADOPTION OR CHILDFREE LIVING

I read of couples wanting advice on when to stop, but our friends and doctors are not stupid enough to jump in front of a speeding train.[1]

When is it time to quit? That's the question couples ask after enduring years of treatment that might include anything from years of temperature charting to multiple in vitro fertilization (IVF) cycles that resulted in no success. Rather than advising them to stop when the money runs out (they could get a loan), or when IVF has failed (they could try again), or when they've spent six years (why not seven?), we've found a different rule of thumb that has proved helpful: *When it hurts more to go on than it does to quit, it's time to quit.*

Many factors may contribute to that hurt that tells infertility patients it's time to quit. Patients may be weary of endless medical appointments, insurance hassles, and needles. They may be financially at the end of their resources. Or they may long for life to return to their pretreatment serenity. They finally want to get off the roller coaster of hope and despair more than they want a biological child.

I've had enough. I can't do this anymore.

We wanted to make sure we were completely done with the IVF so we could move on and not look back. If we're done with this and it still hasn't worked, my wife and I want to change our lives appropriately. Maybe adopt, maybe not—maybe change careers, or do some traveling. I still want children, but when you're running out of options, you have to decide.

Often couples at the early stages of treatment cannot envision a time when they might see adoption or childfree living as preferable to continuing. But part of resolution is that other options begin to look more appealing. The couple whose efforts to conceive have failed must eventually decide between building their family through alternate means (adoption, foster parenting) or spending the rest of their lives together without children.

Adoption: Same Roller Coaster, Different G-Force

Many excellent resources of adoption information are available, and couples considering adoption should avail themselves of these helps. We will include here only a brief explanation of some key terms and some factors to consider when seeking to adopt.

Legally, there are two kinds of adoption—*agency* adoption and *independent* (nonagency or private) adoption. In an agency adoption, the birth parents turn over their parental rights to the agency. In an independent adoption, the birth parents give consent directly to the adoptive parents.

State laws control the adoption process, with four states allowing only agency adoption—Colorado, Connecticut, Delaware, and Massachusetts. More newborns are placed each year through independent adoption than through agency adoption because more birth parents pursue this option.[2] In fact, some 25,000 to 40,000 infants are adopted annually in the United States through private adoption. These numbers exclude foster and relative adoptions, in which the adoptive parents tend to be well acquainted with the birth family's situation.[3]

Children come from two places—within the United States (domestic adoption) and from other countries (international adoption). The number of international adoptions has been going up since the end of World War II. International adoptions currently represent about 10 percent of all U.S. adoptions. In the past ten years, increasing numbers of the children in international adoptions have come from the former Soviet Union and China.[4]

Even when I found we could adopt, I was unsure about opening my heart again. The ache of our losses still lingered, and I knew there were no guarantees. There were so many choices to make and so much red tape to wade through. What if someone decided we wouldn't be good parents? I had my own doubts, after all. We'd already lost three babies through miscarriage, so how could I be sure we were supposed to have children?

My sister and her husband adopted a baby girl, and after several years of treatment, we began to explore adoption. But we decided we just weren't ready for that yet. I was more open to adopting than my husband was, and we wanted to be at the same place about such an important decision.

We've never been at the same place. I wanted treatment, and my wife wanted adoption. Then we'd flip-flop. Then my wife said, "Let's do both because we just don't know." Then this past spring, I wanted to pursue treatment and she didn't think so.

When the time comes that couples have exhausted their medical options and begin to look at the existing choices—adoption or choosing to live without children—they often arrive at that resolution in different timeframes. Often one of the partners—usually, though not always, the wife—would like to pursue adoption but ends up needing to wait for the other spouse to be at the same place. In some ways, this is much like getting engaged in that while both partners are in love, one partner may be ready to commit to marriage before the other is. Applying pressure usually only makes the situation worse.

For several years, I (Sandi) had expressed more interest in adoption than Gary had. And just about the time I thought we were going to end up childfree, he surprised me. We arrived home one evening after attending a wedding, and Gary told me he felt depressed.

"I thought we had a great time. What's wrong?"

"Did you notice how many of our friends attended with their grown children?"

"Yeah."

"For you, babies have been the grief trigger. For me, the pain comes from knowing I'll never go camping with my kid."

"So are you saying you want to adopt?"

"I guess I am."

We checked out U.S. adoption agencies, learning to our surprise that the average cost in our adoption-friendly state was $21,000. Independent adoption is legal in Texas, so we checked out that option because an attorney friend had offered to help us. We attended some adoption seminars and wrote a "Dear Birth Mother" letter in which we described our lives and our values. A few friends helped us distribute the letters to anyone who might come in contact with potential birth parents.

It wasn't long before the calls started coming in from people with possible leads. But we quickly learned not to get our hopes up.

How often do infertile couples hear the words "You can always adopt"—as if it's some easy, instant process. That certainly was not how our experience was turning out.

Through networking with other infertile couples considering adoption, we found that sometimes couples hesitate to pursue adoption out of frustration over having their infertility so minimized by well-meaning friends who offer adoption as an easy solution. The couples we most admired knew that adoption wouldn't solve all the losses they felt; they knew they needed to be at a certain point in resolving their infertility before they pursued adoption, and they knew that the process had its own set of unique stresses.

We found that infertility is not the only process shrouded in a lot of myths. Adoption has its own set of misconceptions:

- Myth: Couples must wait more than five years to get a child.

  Fact: The average wait is actually less than two years.

- Myth: Adoption is very expensive.

  Fact: We agree that adoption should be more affordable. But at this point, it costs about the same as one-and-a-half IVF cycles. Most couples pay around $15,000. The current U.S. $10,000 tax credit helps.

- Myth: Birth parents call all the shots, so they will reject us unless we agree to shared parenting.

  Fact: The law says adoptive families determine the degree of openness. Many experts claim that open adoption—an arrangement in which the birth parent and the child have contact of some sort—is the best option. Little documented evidence exists to support either identified (open) or nonidentified (closed) arrangements. But even in identified adoption arrangements, the adoptive family and birth families may never even meet. Involvement may be as limited as an occasional photo sent through a third party.

- Myth: A lot of couples suffer having a child ripped out of their homes after placement.

  Fact: While this is a truly traumatic experience, it happens in only 1 to 2 percent of all adoptions.

- Myth: Adopted kids have more problems than biological kids.

  Fact: Research shows that adopted children turn out just as well as those raised by their biological parents.

- Myth: Parents who adopt will never love their kids as much as if they had a genetic connection.

Fact: The very institution of marriage demonstrates that you can love as family a person to whom you are not genetically related. Parents who have both biological and adopted children report that the adoptive ties to their children are as strong as their genetic ties.

- Myth: Infertile couples should adopt special-needs children. These couples want kids, and the kids need homes.

  Fact: All of God's children are special creations. But just because special-needs children are available and need parents doesn't mean a particular infertile couple must parent them. Both infertile and fertile couples who consider special-needs children must ask themselves, "Is this the best use of our resources—whether giftedness, financial, temperaments, or support systems?" Some couples are drawn to the unique challenges of raising a child with special needs; others are not. Those who sense no joy at the prospect, who feel no stirring to live sacrificially for a child with special needs, should feel no obligation to do so. For other couples, it is a noble, wonderful pursuit.

Anyone considering adoption needs to know that most agencies and therapists advise couples to finish medical treatment before embarking on the adoption voyage. Despite the misconceptions, the adoption process is stressful. Whereas with infertility treatment, the cycle of hope and despair lasts approximately twenty-eight days, with adoption, the roller coaster has no set times and involves many unexpected twists. Many birth parents do change their minds before placement. The risk of such a change can be decreased, though not eliminated, by working with reputable professionals who provide counseling both for birth parents and for adoptive families.

An additional benefit of working with professionals in the adoption field is that they can provide guidance in helping couples communicate the adoption experience to their children, their families, and their friends. The advice of adoption experts has certainly served us well:

- Avoid phrasing your adoption story with "our daughter *is* adopted." Stating it in the present tense suggests that adoption is ongoing. When it is appropriate to refer to the fact of adoption at all, say, "Our daughter *was* adopted," referring to the way in which she joined your family.
- When people ask if your daughter is your natural child, affirm that she is; the alternative being that she is your *un*natural child!

- Refer to her genetic family as her birth parents. Everyone has birth parents, but not everyone lives in the custody of his or her birth parents.
- When people ask, "Is your daughter one of your own?" tell them, "Certainly." And she is.
- Avoid saying her birth parents relinquished her. Rarely these days is a child abandoned. Today's birth parents do not *surrender* or *release* or *relinquish* or *give up* their child for adoption, except in rare cases of involuntary termination of parental rights due to abuse or neglect. Instead, you can say her birth parents "made an adoption plan." Most birth moms and dads recognize that they are incapable of giving their biological child all that is needed for his or her well-being, so they proactively choose a life for that child that demonstrates selfless love.
- Refer to her adoption as a "domestic adoption." If you have chosen to adopt a child from another country, refer to her adoption as an "international adoption." Formerly this was referred to as *foreign adoption*, but those working in the adoption field pointed out that "foreign" often has negative connotations.
- Describe parents who have chosen to adopt sibling groups, older children, or kids facing particular challenges as parenting "special-needs" children. This is preferable to saying their children were "hard to place." Also, reserve the term "orphan rescue" for cats, dogs, and other animals. The healthiest parents view their adopted special-needs children as blessings, rather than viewing themselves as rescuers.
- When talking about your network of adoptive families, refer to your friends' children who were adopted not as "their adopted children" but simply as "their children." Adoption is one way children join a family, but the modifier "adopted" is unnecessary as an ongoing label. (As adoption expert Patricia Irwin Johnston points out, we would never describe little Jimmy as Tom and Meg's "birth-control-failure child.")

While adoption doesn't "solve" the desire to experience pregnancy and the longing to create a child together, it does fulfill the desire to nurture and parent the next generation.

Each year for the thousands of couples who become adoptive parents, adoption brings resolution to the infertility crisis. That doesn't mean they will forget they were ever infertile. Many of them still detest Mother's Day. Yet the millions of people who join families through adoption, as did Olympic gold-medal winner Scott Hamilton and

Wendy's founder Dave Thomas, are afforded opportunities they never would have had without their adoptive parents.

Going back in time, we see Moses and Esther, members of the Faith Hall of Fame, being raised by adoptive parents—Moses by Pharaoh's daughter, and Esther by her cousin. And the apostle Paul uses adoption as a beautiful metaphor to paint a picture of the believer's relationship with God, our kind Father, once we are rightly related to him through his Son (Rom. 8:23; Gal. 4:5 [NASB]; Eph. 1:5). For those who desire to nurture and raise up the future generation, adoption is both a lovely reality and a fitting picture of how spiritual bonds can be stronger than blood.

Childfree Living: The Road Less Traveled

I decided to go back to school and get a degree in nursing. If I couldn't have a child, I still wanted to nurture and help others.

I may not have children, but I can still leave a lasting legacy.

George Washington fathered no children, but he is called the father of our country. Dr. Seuss had no children, yet he wrote books that have taught millions of kids across several generations to read. Julia Child could just as easily be called Julia Childless. These people and many like them illustrate what Francis Bacon meant when he wrote, "The noblest works and foundations have proceeded from childless men, which have sought to express the images of their minds, where those of their bodies have failed. So the care of posterity is most in them that have no posterity."

We find within the pages of Scripture some couples who had no children. If Priscilla and Aquilla had kids, they go without mention. And the prophetess and judge Deborah appears to have had no children, yet she was called "a mother in Israel" (Judg. 5:7).

A modern example of one who does "noble works" is Mary Beth Lawson. She spends the morning cleaning the home of a housebound church member. Then she heads over to the Pregnancy Resource Center, where she has volunteered for more than a decade. When a friend's teenage daughter got into trouble with the law, the Lawsons opened their home until the girl got her life together. "We wanted children, but that wasn't what God had for us," Mary Beth said. Years after working through the pain of that reality, Mary Beth has chosen to be "Mom" to many young people.

It has been said that there are two kinds of couples without children: those who are childfree by chance and those who are childfree by choice. But there's another group—those who start out in the first group but slowly embrace the second. They begin by calling themselves childless, but eventually they choose to use the label "childfree." These couples are not like those who knew from the start they wouldn't have children. Longing to have kids, they sought medical help, but eventually it became apparent they would not have biological children.

These couples channel their time and energy in other pursuits. Many Christians who do so care for the needs of their church families. Over time they find a place of contentment, seeing the "less" in "childless" emerge as "more."

We now choose to call ourselves "childfree" rather than "childless" because we feel the term childless implies that we're missing something we want—and we no longer are. We consider ourselves childfree. We're free of the loss.

Certainly childfree living is the least understood of the three options for resolving infertility: birth, adoption, and childfree living. Often even other infertile couples cannot comprehend how their friends could choose to live childfree, sometimes even interpreting such a decision as "anti-adoption." Yet many couples who chose childfree living feel adoption is a great fit for their friends; it just doesn't feel right when they try it on themselves. They may decide they'd rather devote their lives to ministry or to other meaningful work.

It may take a while for a couple to become comfortable with this choice. Yet many couples who have done so say they are glad they came to a point of deliberate decision rather than drifting endlessly in indecision. As time passes, they report that the decision feels even more right.

Those who choose to live childfree will encounter some other misconceptions, too.

Myth: Opting to live without kids is unusual.

Fact: The number of childless couples is on the rise; the U.S. Census Bureau estimates that in 1997 more than 35.5 million American couples were childless, either by chance or by choice. That's up by nearly 7 million in a period of twenty years. And demographers expect a 44 percent increase in the number of childless couples by the year 2010. Though the census did not separate the number of those who initially wanted children from those who chose from the start not to have them, the point is that it is becoming more socially acceptable, and less "unusual," to live childfree.

Today about one woman in five between the ages of forty and forty-four is childless. For women that age and younger who have graduate and professional degrees, the figure is 47 percent—nearly half! Some attribute this to women now defining success in terms other than motherhood. Yet when asked to recall their intentions at the time of their last year of college, only 14 percent said that they definitely did not want to have children.[5] Some probably went on to get their advanced degrees *because* they couldn't have kids.

People sometimes ask, "How can you not want children?!" It makes us feel like freaks.

We feel like tweeners. We don't fit anywhere. Going to a new church, where do you have common ground? People our age have a couple of kids. We can hang out with people ten to fifteen years younger. Or we can hang out with empty nesters, people who are fifteen years older.

Those of us without children sometimes wonder if we are really grown-ups.

Myth: Couples without kids are less happy than those with children.

Fact: For all the joys of parenthood, the arrival of a child begins a long drop in marital happiness that hits rock bottom during the child's teen years, according to a national survey. A study of nearly 7,000 spouses shows that couples' pre-baby levels of marital satisfaction return only after all the children have left home. The biggest surprise: childless couples are as happy as couples with children were before the babies arrived. And without the buffeting cycles of childrearing, they tend to stabilize at this high level.[6]

Myth: Childless couples have no one to care for them in their old age, while couples with kids have secure futures.

Fact: Even couples with children have no guarantee their kids will care for them in their old age. Consider the situation of the father who wrote this:

A child came into this world. A boy. "Special needs" is what they labeled him. Never to walk, talk, sing, or dance. He soils himself and relies on the helping hands of others. Some call them diapers. Others call them Depends. I say it depends all right, on who's footing the bill. This child is my son, and although he'll never care for me in my old age, I thank God for his presence. He's taught me more about love and life's challenges than anyone else I've encountered.

None of us knows what tomorrow will bring. Yet concern about preparing for the future is valid. Paul had the care of the aged in mind when he wrote these words: "But if a widow has children or grandchildren, these should learn first of all to put their religion into practice by caring for their own family and so repaying their parents and grandparents, for this is pleasing to God. The widow who is really in need and left all alone puts her hope in God and continues night and day to pray and to ask God for help" (1 Tim. 5:4–5).

As mentioned earlier, in Paul's day, people couldn't buy insurance to provide for future security. Today in the West, couples without children usually have more disposable income and can plan ahead to meet their own future needs.

Leave a Spiritual Legacy

One of the greatest sources of pain for a couple unable to have children is the thought of being unable to leave a legacy. Yet they can leave a spiritual legacy.

I have a question about childlessness. I'd like to know if God might want a couple to be childless to serve him more, for the same reason that God might want a person to be single, to be free to serve him more.

It makes sense, doesn't it? In 1 Corinthians 7, we read about how a single person is more available to serve the Lord than one who is married. In the same way, couples without children have fewer family obligations and the freedom to be more "fruitful," even if they can't "multiply." We see this reflected in the Lord's attitude toward those who never had children, as expressed in Isaiah 56:3–5: "And let not any eunuch complain, 'I am only a dry tree.' For this is what the LORD says: 'To the eunuchs who keep my Sabbaths, who choose what pleases me and hold fast to my covenant—to them I will give within my temple and its walls a memorial and a name better than sons and daughters; I will give them an everlasting name that will not be cut off.'"

A eunuch is a surgically sterilized male. So the eunuch's description of himself as a "dry tree" is a metaphorical reference to his inability to reproduce. In Isaiah's day, "the barbarous practice of self-mutilation and the mutilation of others in this way was prevalent. The law excluded eunuchs from public worship, partly because self-mutilation was often performed in honor of a heathen god, and partly because a maimed creature of any sort was deemed unfit for the service of Yahweh (Lev. 21:16 ff; 22:24)."[7]

Eunuchs were thought to be useless because they had no children. Yet God had a special word of comfort for them: if they developed godly character—if they chose spiritual priorities over material ones—he promised to give them a legacy that would be better than children. What a promise! Such a thing was unheard of. Better than *children*?

We read that they would be memorialized within God's temple. How fitting that centuries after Isaiah penned these words, we see the same ideals lived out in the life of Anna: "There was also a prophetess, Anna, the daughter of Phanuel, of the tribe of Asher. She was very old; she had lived with her husband seven years after her marriage, and then was a widow until she was eighty-four. She never left the temple but worshiped night and day, fasting and praying. Coming up to [Mary and Joseph], . . . she gave thanks to God and spoke about the child to all who were looking forward to the redemption of Jerusalem" (Luke 2:36–38).

Twenty centuries after this childless woman lived, we remember her name—Anna. She served the Lord with her whole being within the temple. And she had the supreme joy of seeing Jesus in his infancy, knowing her Deliverer had finally come.

We learn from this that, as God sees it, spiritual reproduction is even more important than physical reproduction. It has been said that "a person's offspring are his good deeds."

> *If we don't have children, we can be concerned about the neglected children in our assembly. We can put them under our wing in a teaching ministry, or we are free to take the young people to an outing. This can be a great blessing.*
>
> *Motherhood is a blessing, but couples without children are blessed in other ways. We honor motherhood, and we appreciate all our moms have done for us, but we know that fulfillment in life does not hinge on the ability to procreate. God has a plan for us all.*

Though one modern missionary couple, Katarina and John, have no children, they say they now feel far from childless. John said, "We see the young people in our congregation as our very own children. They call us 'Mom' and 'Dad.'"

As Francis Bacon suggested, investing in future generations may take a variety of forms. Those who express the images of their minds through "noble works and foundations" can creatively care for posterity, even though they leave no physical legacy. The apostle Paul, himself childless, had an eternal perspective. And he wrote these fitting words: "For our light and momentary troubles are achieving for us an eternal glory that far outweighs them all. So we fix our eyes not on what is seen, but on what is unseen. For what is seen is temporary, but what is unseen is eternal" (2 Cor. 4:17–18).

DISCUSSION QUESTIONS

1. What part of your infertility is hardest for you to accept and why? Is the same true for your spouse?
2. What are your thoughts on adoption?
3. How do you feel about adopting a child with special needs? Do you and your spouse agree here? Why or why not?
4. Do you sometimes feel "guilted" into considering some adoption scenarios? Why or why not?
5. Does foster parenting appeal to you?
6. What opportunities might you have without children that you would not have with children?
7. When would you say, "Enough is enough," in relation to infertility treatment?
8. Would you and your spouse consider opting to live child-free? What do you see as the main pros and cons for you?

Chapter 21

YOU ARE NOT ALONE

The apostle Paul tells us that all of creation is groaning. My (Sandi's) mother once told me with a sigh that most of life is spent waiting. An infertile friend at church asks me almost weekly, "Please tell me I won't always hurt this much." Life holds many unfulfilled expectations and longings.

During the lecture portion of a monthly infertility support group, a therapist asked the participants how many of them had used drugs. Every single person raised a hand. She then had to clarify that she meant illegal drugs, not fertility drugs. Infertility brings a new way of processing much of life, right down to changing even our perceptions of normal, everyday words. We've said on many occasions that it's a club nobody wants to join. And often after a successful resolution, people assume infertility is over: "You got out—you get to quit the club!" But that's not always the case.

After Dr. Bill placed our daughter, Alexandra, in our arms (by that time, he had resigned from his medical practice and had become our pastor), I knew the pangs of infertility might return on occasion. But I didn't expect to see my current doctor (Dr. Bill's former partner from the same practice) for anything more than annual physicals for a very long time. Yet several years later, I had a positive pregnancy test. This was not the only positive pregnancy test I'd ever had, as you may recall. My body had proven itself a notoriously dangerous place for an embryo. The particular challenge this time, however, was that I'd just flunked my mammogram. So we explored an altogether new question: Should one pursue cancer therapy when pregnant?

As it turned out, we learned two weeks later that the bad spot on the mammogram was from an injury. I'd bruised my sternum with a ski pole. That was the good news. The bad news was that the pregnancy was ectopic (I mentioned this in chapter 18). So I asked my surgeon to tie the other tube while he was removing the ruptured one. That night, Dr. Bill sat with us in "the ditch" until after midnight.

Although I had a sense of finality, in the back of my mind I knew that if doctors someday cured what was wrong with me, I could always bypass the tubes with in vitro fertilization. I never really intended to pursue it, but I found comfort in knowing the door to reproduction wasn't totally shut.

A few years and mission trips later, Dr. Bill resigned from the pastorate and relocated with his family to Kentucky. Sometime after that, I developed some irregular bleeding, so I went again to see my ob-gyn. We tried several hormonal protocols, but nothing worked. Finally, he recommended a uterine ablation, a procedure in which the uterus remains intact but the lining is obliterated.

When I awoke from that procedure, grief came rushing back as the finality set in. *I will never give birth.* At that time I wrote, "I'll *never* know what it looks like to gaze into the face of my biological child. Some days, no biggie. Sometimes like tonight it hurts."

Around that time, Dr. Bill was preparing to fly to Dallas, where we were to do a conference together. I sent him an e-mail to tell him what I was experiencing. He wrote back with this message: "I'm so sorry. There are many different kinds of losses, and this is a very significant one. A bit of teariness is quite fine. I *know* that Gary and Alexandra are wonderful, but don't fill this particular need. Neither do spiritual children, though they are a super thing as well. It's okay to hurt."

That unfulfilled desire is part of why after we wrote our first book on infertility, I decided not to go back and add the good news that Gary and I had adopted Alexandra. We received "the call" two months after the first draft of the manuscript was completed, and we could have added this happy news, but we chose not to. Why? Because we'd had to wrestle with answering "Is God good?" and "Will I trust him?" even if we never had a happy ending.

Some things still remain a mystery, even after "resolution." And there have been new itchings, trials, and longings that have kept us asking the questions about God's goodness and trustworthiness all over again. We'll probably keep asking and answering them until we die.

Yet today we do have a sense of closure and purpose, due in part to continuing opportunities to walk beside those still suffering the pain of being "reproductively challenged." And Dr. Bill has continued to actively minister to infertility patients, having seen the depth of healing and personal growth that can take place when patients have competent medical care that includes compassionate soul care as well. Our desire in writing this book has been to walk with you on an otherwise lonely path, providing companionship from those who have "been there," and by God's grace providing some light that will make it easier for you to keep from stumbling.

Though Gary and I will never have a biological child, we're grateful to have met someone along the way who suggested that infertile couples need two different definitions of success. Of course we dream of that beautiful, biological gift who reflects the ultimate "knowing" of two people in love. Yet there's another kind of success over which we actually have some control . . .

> *I am a success if I get through all this and find that I love*
> *the One who spoke the stars into being*
> *even more than I did when I started,*
> *though at times it has felt like I've walked alone on starless nights.*

> *I am a success if I've managed to keep from shutting out*
> *my most important relationships,*
> *choosing instead to tenaciously initiate intimacy*
> *even when I've had no strength left of my own with which to knock on*
>   *the door.*

> *I am a success if I've allowed these treacherous rapids to cut*
> *canyons of inner beauty as I'm shaped,*
> *unable to resist, careening along,*
> *letting go of control and learning instead to trust.*

> *I am a success if I've made righteous decisions*
> *yet express true empathy for those who have chosen different courses,*
> *wiping their tears with my thumb*
> *when they have faced consequences from their choices.*

> *I am a success if, in the midst of these endless, intense longings,*
> *I still dance in the shadows on a silent floor,*
> *hoping beyond reason because earthquakes and darkness*
> *sometimes suggest an imminent resurrection.*

You are not alone!

WORKBOOK

EXERCISES FOR COUPLES

Exercise 1: Marriage

1. Read Genesis 2:18–22 and Genesis 3:18. What are some differences between the man and the woman?
2. Based on Genesis 1:26–31 and 2:23–25, what are some ways in which the man and the woman are similar?
3. Based on Genesis 2:24, in what way are the man and woman united and interdependent?
4. In what way are you and your spouse different? In what ways are you alike? How are you interdependent and united?
5. Describe your similarities and differences as you face infertility. How can you function more as one?
6. Read 1 Peter 2:21–3:12.
   a. According to 2:22–23, what did Jesus do when people were rude and insulting to him?
   b. How can you be like Jesus in your responses to people's senseless remarks?
   c. For her: According to 3:1–6, what is precious to God?
   d. For him: According to 3:7, what should your response to your wife look like?
   e. For both: If your marriage were like the relationship described in 3:8–12, what would be different? What steps can you take together to improve your harmony?
   f. Join hands and pray silently together, thanking God for each other and asking him to strengthen your relationship.

For further reading on gender differences: Elaine Storkey. *Origins of Difference: The Gender Debate Revisited.* Grand Rapids: Baker, 2001.

Exercise 2: Communication

Research tells us that the following four communication styles are especially deadly in the marriage relationship.[1]

Withdrawal. One partner hides behind the paper, purposely avoiding the other, or even gets up to make a sandwich to ignore what's being said. This is the most damaging of the four patterns.

Escalation. What starts out as minor conflict over the trash ends up as World War III, punctuated with, "And your mother's ugly, too!"

Negative Interpretation. "No good deed goes unpunished!" One says something that's intended to be positive, or at least neutral, and the other partner interprets it as being selfish or unkind.

Invalidation. A person and his or her opinions are treated as if they are of no consequence. This communicates, "Not only are your thoughts worthless, but so are *you*."

1. Which of these communication styles do you most often resort to?
2. Which of these is more characteristic of your partner?
3. What are some steps the two of you can take to replace these unhealthy patterns with more constructive communication patterns?
4. Answer the following true or false:
   a. My partner listens well.
   b. My partner understands how I feel.
   c. We creatively handle our differences.
   d. We have a hard time making financial decisions.
   e. We have a good balance of leisure time spent together and apart.
   f. It's easy to come up with activities to do together.
   g. I am satisfied with how we talk to each other.
   h. Our sexual relationship is fulfilling.
   i. I can share my feelings during disagreements.
   j. My partner understands my opinions and ideas.

Now go back and indicate how you think your spouse would answer these questions. Discuss your responses.

5. Determine your top needs.
   a. List what you consider your five greatest needs in your marriage relationship.
   b. List what you think your spouse would say are his or her greatest needs.

    c.   Compare answers. Were you close? Why or why not?

    d.   How can you better meet each other's needs?

Exercise 3: Sexual Intimacy

A study presented by Dr. Jennifer Norten at a conference of the American Society for Reproductive Medicine (ASRM) determined the following: "Women undergoing infertility treatment experience significant changes in various aspects of sexual desire, arousal, orgasm, length of foreplay, and frequency of intercourse."[2]

1.   Has your own experience been similar to this?
2.   Would your spouse say this finding reflects his or her experience?
3.   What are some ways you can bring new vitality to your sexual relationship?

Following are some discussion questions that we hope will help you find deeper satisfaction in your sex life. They have been excerpted and adapted from our book *Sexual Intimacy in Marriage*. The greatest sexual problem is the inability to talk about sex. The topics below are designed to help you explore details of your intimate life together and to enhance your times of lovemaking sex, not baby-making sex. We strongly recommend that you discuss these questions outside of the context of lovemaking. If you think of other questions you'd like to talk about, add them.

- What time of day are you usually together sexually?
- Is this the optimum time for both partners?
- Where does it usually happen?
- Where would you like it to happen?
- What degree of lighting do you usually have?
- What variety in lighting would you like to try?
- Do hygiene issues ever inhibit your desire?
- Does one of you usually initiate more than the other? Is this the way you both want it?
- What are your unspoken signals that say "I'm interested"?
- Are there other ways you'd like to communicate interest? Other ways you'd like your spouse to let you know that he or she is interested?
- What do you usually wear?
- How long does it usually take for her from excitation to ultimate satisfaction?
- How long does it usually take for him from excitation to ultimate satisfaction?

- How do you want to be pursued? Hint and then back off? Hint and then try again in a different way? Hint and go for it? Never mind the hints—just go for it? Other?
- How do you want to be told to do something differently? Discussion outside of sex? Gentle redirecting of hands? Verbally?
- How do you generally redirect your partner? How does he or she feel about that?
- What kinds of caresses do you prefer? On what parts of the body? *With* what parts of the body?
- What positions increase excitement for you? What sustains desire? What decreases your interest?
- Do you have any uncommunicated fantasies? Strip Monopoly? Showering together? Polaroids or digital photos of each other?
- Discuss the degree of dress or undress that arouses you.
- Discuss the kind and color of apparel you like. (A husband may not care for black negligees, but his wife has been wearing them for years; or a husband may give his wife an annual Valentine's Day Frederick's of Hollywood corset, which she dislikes.)
- Are you courageous enough to walk into a lingerie department and buy something *you* would like to enjoy seeing on your spouse?
- How can you draw the five senses (sight, touch, smell, taste, sound) into your lovemaking?
- Interact with this statement: "We're totally comfortable being naked together, but the surprise and delight of seeing each other nude no longer brings the erotic rush it did when we were first married." Is this true for you? Why or why not? What are the advantages and disadvantages to mature, time-honored love?
- What sets the mood for him? For her?
- How much do you want left to the imagination?
- What elements enhance the whole experience for you?
- List an assortment of ideal atmospheres you'd like to try.
- What changes have taken place in your sex life since beginning your infertility workup?
- What could you do to improve your intimate time together?

Exercise 4: Reducing Stress

Do calming exercises. Some experts recommend reducing anxiety and stress through relaxation techniques such as deep breathing or meditating for five minutes. While Eastern meditation involves emptying the mind, Christian meditation involves filling the mind with Scripture and ruminating on truth. Relaxation may not cure infertility, but it certainly won't impair it!

Step 1: Pick a Scripture you know, such as the Lord's Prayer or Psalm 23.

Step 2: Sit quietly in a comfortable position.

Step 3: Close your eyes.

Step 4: Relax your muscles.

Step 5: Breathe slowly and naturally. Inhale slowly counting to six, then exhale for a slow count of six. Use your diaphragm, not just your chest, and as you do, mentally recite Scripture or imagine a lovely scene.

Step 6: Assume a passive attitude. Don't worry about how well you're doing. When other thoughts come to mind, simply return to your original focus.

Exercise 5: Assisting Your Doctor

Complete the worksheet on pages 262–63. It's not exhaustive, nor does every patient need every test. And the order in which you complete these tests will vary. You can save time and increase accuracy by keeping track of tests, results, and dates, and having the information handy when you go to the doctor's office or call with a question.

Keep a calendar of all the medications you've taken and the dosages, including for the HCG shot, period flow, spotting, and any other symptoms. If you need to call your doctor (or his or her partner) during evenings or weekends, your medical team won't have access to this information, and having it available at such times can be important.

Exercise 6: Discussing Adoption

1. Erma Bombeck was an adoptive parent. Read below what she wrote on motherhood. Then talk about your view of a "real" parent.

   You want to know what "real" is?
   Real is what gets a part-time job to pay for a baton that lights up.
   Real is what hears, "I hate you" and still says "No."
   Real is what sits up until 3 AM when she has the car out and it's raining.
   Real is hurting when she's in pain and laughing when she's happy.

INFERTILITY WORKUP WORKSHEET

Test	Date	Results	Retest Date	Results	Retest Date	Results
Semenalysis						
Postcoital Test						
Ovulation						
LH sticks						
Serial Sonography						
Progesterone Level						
Endometrial Biopsy						
Hormonal						
Estrogen						
Progesterone						
Prolactin						
Androgens						
Testosterone						

	Date	Results
DHEA-S		
Thyroid		
Other		
Anatomy		
Sonography		
HSG		
Laparoscopy		
Tubal Irrigation		
Hysteroscopy		
Immunological Tests		
Genetic Tests		
Husband		
Wife		

Real is emergency rooms, PTAs, music that deafens, lies,
    defiance, and slammed doors.
Real is what shows up every day![3]

2. Discuss these questions:

    •   Do I feel I can love a child who looks nothing like me, a child
        who doesn't resemble anything about me, including my
        mannerisms and the way I walk?
    •   What will I do if my child turns out to have a significantly
        disabling condition after the adoption has been finalized?
    •   If my child decided to search for his or her birth parent(s),
        would I assist and support him or her in that process?

Exercise 7: Discussing Childfree Living

Living without children doesn't necessarily mean you can't relate
to kids. In addition to Dr. Seuss's Grinch and Cindy Lou Who, characters such as Mary Poppins, Peter Pan, and Alice in Wonderland were
created by people who were childfree. And six U.S. presidents fathered
no children: George Washington, James Madison, Andrew Jackson,
James Buchanan, Warren Harding, and James Polk.

Discuss the following:

1. Even though our bodies have not cooperated to create a child,
    what else might we create together that would be uniquely "us"?
2. We often focus on the biblical command to be fruitful and on
    God's creation of woman as man's "helper," and we think
    godly women must be wives and mothers. But God also gave
    the man and woman dominion over the earth. What are some
    ways to exercise dominion in a way that benefits the earth and
    its creatures?
3. If we choose to resolve our infertility by living childfree, what are
    some ways that appeal to us for investing in future generations?
4. What steps do we need to take financially to assure that, to the
    best of our ability, we've taken care of our future health-care
    needs?
5. For whom can we be spiritual parents?
6. How can we use the advantages of our situation to invest in eter-
    nal pursuits, such as giving sacrificially, doing volunteer work,
    traveling to do short-term mission work, opening our home to
    the disadvantaged, or doing occupational ministry in a place
    that might be too dangerous for children?

Appendix 2

CHRISTIAN MEDICAL ASSOCIATION STATEMENT ON REPRODUCTIVE TECHNOLOGY

Preamble

The family is the basic social unit as designed by God. It is formed as a man and woman make an exclusive marital commitment for love, companionship, intimacy, and spiritual union. As a result of their physical union, children may be added to the family.

Children are a gift and responsibility from God to the family. Parents are entrusted with providing and modeling love, nurture, protection, and spiritual training. The inability to have children need not diminish the fullness of the family.

Infertile couples may choose adoption or seek medical care when they desire children. Adoption emulates God's adoption of us as spiritual children. Some reproductive technologies are an appropriate exercise of mankind's God-given creativity.

Certain reproductive technologies may present direct and indirect dangers to the family. As technology permits further divergence from normal physiologic reproduction, it increasingly leads to perplexing moral dilemmas. Not every technological procedure may be morally justified.

The principles which can guide the development and implementation of reproductive technologies include the following: First, conception resulting from the union of a wife's egg and her husband's sperm is the biblical design. Second, individual human life begins at conception; therefore, God intends for us to protect it. Third, God holds us morally responsible for our genetic offspring.

Statement

CMDA approves the following procedures as consistent with God's design for the family:

- Education about fertilization
- Medical treatment (e.g., ovulation-inducing drugs)
- Surgical intervention (e.g., for anatomic abnormalities hindering fertility)
- Artificial insemination by husband (AIH)
- Adoption
- In vitro fertilization (IVF) with husband's sperm and wife's egg, with subsequent:
  a. Transfer to uterus (ER-embryo replacement)
  b. Zygote intrafallopian transfer (ZIFT)

- Gamete intrafallopian transfer (GIFT)—Husband's sperm and wife's egg
- Cryopreservation of sperm or egg

CMDA cannot speak with certainty about the place of the following procedures in God's design for the family:

- Artificial insemination by donor (AID)
- In vitro fertilization (donor egg or donor sperm)
- Gamete intrafallopian transfer (donor egg or donor sperm)
- Zygote intrafallopian transfer (donor egg or donor sperm)

  Reason: While there is no clear biblical support for the concept of the introduction of a third party, there is strong biblical support for the ideal of a family as defined in the preamble of this statement.

- Cryopreservation of embryos with specific safeguards

  Reason: Cryopreservation raises the possibility of embryo destruction and preservation of excessive embryos.

CMDA opposes the following procedures as inconsistent with God's design for the family:

- Selective abortion for embryo reduction or sex selection
- Surrogate mother procedures
- Transfer of excessive numbers of embryos to a recipient mother
- Uterine lavage for embryo transfer
- Discarding of embryos
- Non-therapeutic experimentation with embryos

Conclusion

CMDA affirms the need for continued moral scrutiny of our developing reproductive technology as it impacts the family. We recognize that as physicians we must use our creative capacity within the limits of God's design. Couples who suffer from infertility should be encouraged to seek pastoral guidance and counsel, as well as to pray for God's wisdom in the use of these technologies.

Addendum

In this statement, embryo refers to the conceptus from the moment of fertilization. We do not differentiate between the new term "pre-embryo" and embryo.

Guidelines for Cryopreservation of Embryos:

1. Cryopreservation of embryos should be done with the sole intent of future transfer to the genetic mother.
2. Embryos should be produced from the husband's sperm and the wife's eggs.
3. A limited number of embryos should be produced to eliminate cryopreservation of excessive numbers of embryos.
4. There should be pre-agreement on the part of the couple that if the wife becomes pregnant, all remaining frozen embryos will be transferred back into her at future times of her choice.
5. There should also be pre-agreement that in a situation in which the embryos cannot be transferred to the wife (e.g., where the wife dies or has a hysterectomy) they will be adopted by another couple who desire to have a child for themselves by having the embryos transferred to the adoptive mother.

Approved by the CMDA House of Delegates
Passed with a vote of 63 for, 1 opposed
May 3, 1990
Toronto, Canada

Glossary

Ablation. See endometrial ablation.

Adhesion. Adjacent tissues sticking to one another. They can be thin and filmy like plastic wrap or thick, tenacious, and difficult to divide. Adhesions in the abdominal cavity, fallopian tubes, or inside the uterus can interfere with the egg's movement and implantation of the embryo.

Amenorrhea. The absence or abnormal cessation of menstruation.

Ampule. A glass vessel used to hold solution for injection.

Analog. A chemical compound that is structurally similar to another but differs slightly in composition

Androgens. Hormones that cause masculine type changes such as oily skin, facial hair, and weight gain. When elevated, may lead to fertility problems in both men and women.

Antibodies. Proteins made by the body to fight or attack foreign substances entering the body. Normally, antibodies prevent infection, but sometimes they attack gametes or embryos, causing infertility.

Artificial insemination. The process of depositing sperm at the cervix or directly into the uterus (intrauterine insemination, IUI), with the use of a syringe.

ARTs (assisted reproductive technologies). According to the broadest definition (which we use), ARTs are procedures used to bring about conception without sexual intercourse (such as IUI, IVF, ICSI, and ZIFT). A more limited definition would include only those procedures that involve the handling of eggs and sperm.

ASRM. The American Society for Reproductive Medicine.

Assisted hatching. The use of mechanical or chemical thinning of the outer shell of a fertilized egg prior to embryo transfer to enhance the embryo's ability to more easily divide and implant after transfer.

Autonomy. The ethical principle of allowing a human being self-directing freedom or moral independence. In the context of medical treatment, this means the patient has the right to make decisions about care rendered to him or her.

Azoospermia. The absence of sperm in the seminal fluid.

Basal body temperature (BBT). The body temperature when taken at its lowest point, usually in the morning before getting out of bed. Charting one's BBT is used to predict ovulation.

Beneficence. The ethical principle of "Do good." An action is determined to be beneficent if the reason for doing it is to bring about a good goal.

Beta HCG test (Beta human chorionic gonadotropin test). A blood test given to detect the presence of an early pregnancy and to monitor embryo development.

Biochemical pregnancy. A pregnancy initially determined to be positive via measuring the blood serum HCG (human chorionic gonadotropin) level but that turned negative because the embryo stopped growing.

Bioethics. The morality of health care.

Blastocyst. An early stage of embryo development (reached approximately five days after fertilization). The blastocyst looks like a hollow ball of cells with a secondary cluster of cells on the inner wall at one end. The inner group of cells will develop into the baby, while the outer sphere becomes the supporting structures such as placenta and amniotic sac.

"Blighted ovum." A so-called blighted ovum occurs when the placental portion of the pregnancy develops but the fetus does not. Using the term "blighted ovum" is both sexist and inaccurate, as it blames the female (ovum), when technically, once fertilized, it isn't an ovum any longer; it's a zygote. Whether or not it develops properly may be related to sperm, egg, or both. "Early miscarriage" is a more appropriate term.

Cervix. The lower portion of the uterus that extends into the vagina.

Cervical mucus. A substance that plugs the opening of the cervix. Usually it prevents sperm and bacteria from entering the womb, but at ovulation, under the influence of estrogen, the mucus becomes thin, watery, and stretchy to allow sperm to pass.

Chlamydia. A sexually transmitted disease that is often without symptoms. Left untreated, it can cause infertility both through pelvic inflammatory disease and ectopic pregnancy.

Chromosome. The structure in the cell that carries the genes. Humans have forty-six chromosomes, with half coming from the egg and half from the sperm. At conception, a human life has all the chromosomes it will ever have.

Chromopertubation. The process of injecting colored dye through the fallopian tubes and observing through a laparoscope to determine if the tubes are open or blocked.

Cilia. Small hairlike projections that line the inside of the fallopian tubes. Their wavelike action carries the egg toward the uterus.

Clitoris. The sex organ of the female that has no other function than to provide sexual pleasure. It contains an enormous number of sensory nerves and in terms of sexual sensation is the female counterpart to the head of the penis.

Clomid. Clomiphene citrate (also Serophene and Milophene). A fertility drug that stimulates the release of gonadotropins from the pituitary gland.

Cloning. A procedure in which an individual is grown from a single somatic cell of its parent and is genetically identical to that parent or gene donor.

"Compassionate" transfer. Embryo transfer done at a time in the menstrual cycle that is unlikely to support a pregnancy, using thawed embryos that were cryopreserved.

Conception. Used by many to refer to the moment when sperm fertilizes an egg and when DNA aligns (as in the case of cloning), resulting in the creation of a unique human being. Howerver, since 1972, medical dictionaries have defined conception as the time at which an embryo implants in the uterus, an event that happens well after fertilization.

Corpus luteum. The hormone-producing structure resulting from ovulation of a mature follicle. Yellow in appearance, it is essential for the normal production of progesterone. Progesterone causes the slight rise in basal temperature that happens at the midpoint of the menstrual cycle. If the corpus luteum does not function as it should, the uterine lining may fail to support a pregnancy. Once fertilization occurs, the corpus luteum maintains the uterine lining, supporting the implanted embryo. If the corpus luteum fails to produce progesterone for long enough or in sufficient quantities, the endometrium is unable to sustain a pregnancy. This is called a luteal phase defect (LPD).

Cryopreservation. Freezing a human embryo at supercold temperatures, which puts it in suspended animation, a state in which it can retain its viability for an undetermined length of time.

Danazol. A medication occasionally used to treat endometriosis. It suppresses the production of luteinizing hormone (LH) and follicle-stimulating hormone (FSH) by the pituitary and causes a state of amenorrhea, during which the endometrial implants (endometriosis) waste away. Many women experience oily skin, acne, weight gain, abnormal hair growth, deepening of the voice, and muscle cramps with this medication.

Danocrine. See Danazol.

DE. See donor egg.

DES (diethylstilbestrol). A medication prescribed for several decades to prevent miscarriage. Fetuses exposed in utero to this drug developed numerous problems, including cancer, deformities, and infertility. DES is no longer prescribed for this indication but may be useful prior to conception for improving cervical mucus.

DHEA-S (dehydroepiandrosterone sulfate). Also DHEA-sulfate. See androgens.

DI. See donor insemination.

DNA (deoxyribonucleic acid). The molecular basis of heredity that makes up the genes, within the chromosomes, which determine all of a person's physical characteristics.

Donor egg (DE). Ovum (or plural, ova) provided by the genetic rather than the biological or "birth" mother. Also refers to the procedure by which an egg from a female donor is mixed with sperm to create an embryo, which is then transferred to the uterus of the woman who will carry it to term (the gestational carrier).

Donor insemination (DI). Artificial insemination using sperm from a donor rather than from the husband. Sperm is deposited at the cervix or directly into the uterus (intrauterine insemination, IUI), using a syringe.

Ectopic pregnancy. A potentially life-threatening situation in which pregnancy takes place outside of the uterus, usually in a fallopian tube.

Egg donation. See donor egg.

Egg retrieval. Also called egg harvest. A procedure used (often following superovulation) to obtain eggs from ovarian follicles for use in in vitro fertilization. The procedure may be performed by laparoscopy or by using a transvaginal sonographically guided needle to locate the follicle within the ovary.

Ejaculate. (n.) Semen released during male orgasm.

Embryo. A human life in its earliest form. An embryo is formed when egg and sperm unite, followed within twenty-four hours by the alignment of their DNA.

Embryo adoption. The release of one's "leftover" cryopreserved embryos for adoption by another (usually infertile) couple. Or from the other side, the process of receiving for thaw and transfer the frozen embryos from another couple. This process often involves a home study and legal agreements.

Embryo donation. Another term for embryo adoption.

Embryo transfer (ET). The process of placing an egg that was fertilized outside of the womb into a woman's fallopian tube or uterus. Often ET appears in conjunction with in vitro fertilization (IVF) as IVF-ET.

Embryologist. A person specializing in the scientific study of embryo development.

Endometrial ablation. An outpatient surgical procedure to eliminate or reduce bleeding from the uterus by destroying the uterine lining, using heated fluid, electrocautery, or various types of laser.

Endometrial biopsy. A procedure in which the physician collects a sample of the uterine lining for analysis. The biopsy results can confirm ovulation and the proper preparation of the endometrium for implantation.

Endometriosis. A condition in which endometrial tissue forms outside the uterus, sometimes causing pain and infertility.

Endometrium. The lining of the uterus, which grows and sheds in response to hormonal stimulation; the tissue designed to nourish the implanted embryo.

Endorphins. Natural narcotics manufactured in the brain to reduce sensitivity to pain and stress. The body produces endorphins in response to orgasm, exercise, laughter, chocolate, and chili peppers.

Erection. The process during which the penis becomes engorged with blood, causing it to swell and become rigid.

Estrogen. A group of hormones that causes feminizing changes such as fatty deposits on the breasts and hips, higher voice, lack of facial hair.

ET. See embryo transfer.

Fertilization. The process in which the sperm penetrates the egg, resulting in a human embryo when the chromosomes align and activate.

Fertiloscope. A small needlelike scope that goes through the back wall of the vagina into the pelvic cavity. Slightly larger than a large-bore needle, it can be used in the doctor's office in conjunction with local anesthesia. Saline is injected, allowing the operator to examine parts of the pelvis and ovaries that fall naturally into view. If no adhesions are present, the doctor can see the back of the uterus, the ovaries, and sometimes even into the ends of the fallopian tubes.

Fertinorm HP. A highly purified preparation of follicle-stimulating hormone (FSH), a gonadotropin. Its principal action is the induction of follicular growth in infertile women who do not have primary ovarian failure.

Fimbria. Tiny fingerlike projections at the entrance of the fallopian tubes.

Follicle. Fluid-filled sac in the ovary that contains the egg to be released at ovulation.

Follicular phase. The portion of a woman's cycle prior to ovulation (usually between seven and twenty-one days) during which a follicle grows and high levels of estrogen cause the lining of the uterus to proliferate.

FSH (follicle-stimulating hormone). A pituitary hormone that stimulates sperm development in the male and follicular development in the female. In both men and woman, elevated levels of this hormone indicate gonadal failure. Brand names include Gonal F, Fertinex, Follistim, and Bravelle.

Gamete. A reproductive cell—sperm in the man, ovum (or egg) in the woman.

General revelation. What God reveals about himself through nature and the world at large.

Gestation. The carrying of a life within the uterus.

Gestational surrogacy. A third-party reproduction arrangement in which a woman carries to term an embryo to which she is not genetically related.

GIFT (gamete intrafallopian transfer). A procedure in which, following egg retrieval, sperm and eggs are mixed and injected into the fallopian tubes, allowing fertilization to take place in its natural environment.

Glucophage. Brand name for metformin, a medication that lowers blood sugar by keeping the liver from making too much sugar. Used in infertility treatment for patients with polycystic ovarian syndrome (PCOS).

Gonadotropin-releasing hormone (GnRH; also GnRHa, for Gonadotropin-releasing hormone agonist). A hormone secreted by the hypothalamus approximately every ninety minutes, enabling the pituitary to secrete gonadotropins, such as luteinizing hormone (LH) and follicle-stimulating hormone (FSH), which stimulate the gonads. See also FSH and LH. Brand names of GnRH agonists include Lupron, Zoladex, and Synarel.

Gonads. The glands (testicles, ovaries) that make reproductive cells (sperm, ova) and sex hormones (testosterone, estrogen).

GnRH. See gonadotropin-releasing hormone.

GnRHa. Gonadotropin-releasing hormone agonist.

GnRHa analog. Medication that works like a gonadotropin-releasing hormone. It results in an initial stimulation of the pituitary followed by a prolonged suppression of pituitary hormones. It is often used to shut down the natural menstrual cycle before beginning a cycle using assisted reproductive technologies. See Lupron.

HCG (human chorionic gonadotropin). A hormone produced in early pregnancy that signals the corpus luteum to keep producing progesterone. HCG is also injected to trigger ovulation in women and is used to stimulate testosterone production in men. Brand names include Ovidrel, Novarel, Pregnyl, and Profasi.

Heterotopic gestation. A pregnancy in which at least two embryos are present, one being in the uterus and one outside the uterus (ectopic).

HMG (human menopausal gonadotropin). A combination of hormones (LH and FSH) used to induce ovulation in a variety of fertility treatments. (Historically, HMG was collected and purified from the urine of nuns.) Brand names include Pergonal and Repronex.

Host uterus. Also called a "surrogate gestational mother." A couple's embryo is transferred to the uterus of another woman (the "host") who carries the pregnancy to term, having agreed to give the baby to the genetic parents immediately after birth.

HSG. See hysterosalpingogram.

Huhner's test. Also called postcoital test (PCT) or Sims-Huhner test. A microscopic examination of the cervical mucus best performed within two hours after intercourse to determine compatibility between the woman's mucus and the man's semen. This test is used to detect sperm-mucus interaction problems and the presence of sperm antibodies and to assess the quality of cervical mucus.

Human papillomavirus (HPV). A sexually transmitted disease (STD) that can cause infertility if untreated.

Hyperstimulation. Also called superovulation. The use of fertility drugs to stimulate the ovary to produce multiple eggs.

Hyperthyroidism. The overproduction of hormones by the thyroid gland.

Hypothalamus. The brain's hormone regulation center.

Hypothyroidism. The underproduction of hormones by the thyroid gland.

Hysterosalpingogram (HSG). A procedure in which dye is injected through the vagina and cervix into the uterus. Once the uterine cavity fills with the dye, if the fallopian tubes are open, the fluid spills into the abdominal cavity. X-ray images may indicate if the tubes are blocked and, if so, where. Uterine cavity shape and presence of polyps or fibroids can also be determined.

Hysteroscopy. A procedure in which the doctor inserts a fiber-optic scope into the uterus to check for abnormalities. Minor surgical repairs can sometimes be done during this procedure.

ICSI (intracytoplasmic sperm injection). A micromanipulation procedure in which a single sperm is injected into the egg. This sometimes allows for fertilization even in the case of low sperm count or nonmotile sperm.

Implantation. The embedding of the embryo into the tissue of the uterine wall so it can establish contact with the mother's blood supply. Implantation ideally occurs in the lining of the uterus; in an ectopic pregnancy, however, implantation occurs outside the uterus.

Infertility, primary. The inability to conceive after one year of unprotected intercourse and/or the inability to carry a pregnancy to term.

Infertility, secondary. The inability to conceive or carry to term after having had one or more children.

Infertility workup. Initial medical examinations and tests done to determine the cause(s) of infertility.

Intrafallopian. Within the fallopian tubes.

Intracytoplasmic sperm injection. See ICSI.

IUI (intrauterine insemination). A doctor uses a catheter to place specially treated sperm directly into a woman's uterus.

IVF-ET (in vitro fertilization–embryo transfer). The process of surgically removing eggs from a woman (often following superovulation), mixing the eggs with sperm in a culture dish in the laboratory, and later transferring the embryo(s) to the uterus.

Justice. In the context of reproductive ethics, justice is the ethical principle of equitable administration of the law and a human being's individual rights.

Laparoscopy. A procedure in which a small telescope is inserted into an incision in the abdominal wall to view the internal organs. This allows diagnosis and treatment of a number of fertility problems, including endometriosis, abdominal adhesions, and polycystic ovaries. Laparoscopy is also used by some clinics in egg retrieval for IVF (in vitro fertilization) and with GIFT (gamete intrafallopian transfer) and ZIFT (zygote intrafallopian transfer) procedures.

Levirate marriage. Old Testament law that required the surviving brother-in-law (or the nearest male relative) to marry his deceased brother's widow and impregnate her. The firstborn son resulting from their union was named for the deceased, allowing his name to be carried on.

LH (luteinizing hormone). A pituitary hormone that stimulates the gonads. LH is necessary for sperm and testosterone production in males and for estrogen production in females. When estrogen reaches its peak, the pituitary releases a surge of LH, which releases the egg from the follicle.

Lupron. A brand name for leuprolide acetate. A long-acting GnRH analog. An injection of Lupron results in an initial stimulation of the pituitary followed by a prolonged suppression of pituitary hormones. Since Lupron lowers estrogen levels, it is an effective treatment for endometriosis, though it has never been approved by the FDA for this purpose. It is often used to shut down the natural menstrual cycle before beginning a cycle using assisted reproductive technologies. Lupron, Lupron Depot, Lupron Depot-Ped, and Viadur are each synthetic analogs of naturally occurring gonadotropin-releasing hormone (Gn- or LH-releasing hormones). The analog possesses greater potency than the natural hormone.

Luteal phase. The postovulatory phase, or second half, of a woman's cycle. During this phase, the corpus luteum produces progesterone, making the uterine lining thicker so it can support the implantation and growth of the embryo.

Luteal phase defect (LPD). A deficiency in the amount of progesterone produced (or in the length of time it is produced) by the corpus luteum. An LPD can render the endometrium unable to sustain a pregnancy.

Luteinizing hormone. See LH.

Male-factor infertility. Infertility in which a male factor is the cause or a contributing cause.

Masturbation. Manual stimulation of the sex organ, leading to orgasm. Male masturbation is used to collect semen for analysis and for artificial insemination.

Menstruation. The female's cyclical shedding of the uterine lining in response to stimulation from estrogen and progesterone.

MESA (microscopic epididymal sperm aspiration). The process of harvesting immature sperm by needle aspiration of the existing ductwork, then using micromanipulation for fertilization.

Metphormin. Medication that lowers blood sugar by keeping the liver from making too much sugar. Used in infertility treatment for patients with polycystic ovarian syndrome (PCOS). Brand name: Glucophage.

Methotrexate. In the context of infertility, methotrexate is a chemotherapy (chemical agent) drug used in the nonsurgical treatment of ectopic pregnancy.

Metrodin. Pure FSH (follicle-stimulating hormone) in injectable form used to stimulate ovulation.

Micromanipulation. Procedures in which fertilization is induced by various methods designed for overcoming infertility. These techniques involve securing or "stabilizing" a harvested egg under the microscope with a special glass instrument and then piercing the egg with a tiny glass "needle" before injecting a single sperm. Micromanipulation also includes "assisted hatching," the use of mechanical or chemical thinning of the outer shell of a fertilized egg prior to embryo transfer to enhance the embryo's ability to more easily divide and implant after transfer.

Milophene. One brand name for clomiphene citrate, a fertility drug that stimulates the release of gonadotropins from the pituitary gland.

Miscarriage. Spontaneous pregnancy loss occurring within the first twenty weeks of pregnancy.

Morphology. In the context of infertility treatment, the study of the structure of sperm to determine the number or percentage of sperm in a sample that appear to have been formed normally. Sperm that are structured abnormally are kinked or have double heads or coiled tails.

Motile. Exhibiting or capable of movement.

Motility. Sperm movement properties, including the ability to propel in a forward direction.

Multifetal pregnancy reduction. The destruction of one or more fetuses in a multiple gestation resulting from an in vitro fertilization (IVF) procedure. The goal is usually to improve the chances of survival for the remaining embryos, though sometimes it is done to reduce a pregnancy to one embryo when only one child is desired.

Nonmaleficence. The ethical principle of "Do no harm."

Nucleus of egg. A central structure within the egg that contains the DNA material.

One-flesh principle. An ethical principle—derived from but not stated in the Bible—that says gametes may be united only when they are from a man and a women who are married to each other.

Oocyte. An egg before maturation.

Orgasm. The psychological and physical thrill that accompanies sexual climax.

Ovulation. The release of the mature egg (ovum) from an ovarian follicle.

Ovulation induction. Treatment performed using medication to initiate, or induce, ovulation.

Ovum donation. See egg donation.

Pituitary gland. The body's master hormonal gland that extends from the base of the brain and is stimulated by the hypothalamus. The pituitary controls all hormonal functions.

Pergonal. A brand name for human menopausal gonadotropin (HMG). Medication used to replace the pituitary hormones (luteinizing hormone and follicle-stimulating hormone). It is used to induce ovulation in women and to stimulate sperm production in men.

Polycystic ovarian syndrome (PCOS). Also called Stein-Leventhal syndrome. A condition found in women who don't ovulate regularly, if at all. Characterized by excessive production of male sex hormones (androgens) and the presence of cysts in the ovaries.

Postcoital test (PCT). Also called Huhner's test or Sims-Huhner test. A microscopic examination of the cervical mucus best performed within two hours after intercourse to determine compatibility between a woman's mucus and the man's semen. This test is used to detect sperm-mucus interaction problems and the presence of sperm antibodies and to assess the quality of cervical mucus.

Pre-embryo. An ill-defined term sometimes applied to the embryo in the first ten to fourteen days following fertilization.

Preimplantation genetic diagnosis (PGD). A procedure whereby an embryo can be tested for genetic or chromosomal abnormalities before transfer to the uterus. Embryos found to be carriers of genetic disorders are discarded, and only embryos deemed healthy are transferred. For those who consider the human embryo to have the full rights of personhood, this procedure is deemed unethical.

Premature ovarian failure. A condition in which the ovary runs out of follicles before the normal age associated with menopause (forty-five to fifty-two years, on average). Primitive germ cells ultimately provide the 1 to 2 million oocytes that are present in the ovaries at birth. This number is reduced at puberty through cell death to approximately 300,000.

Progesterone. The female sex hormone secreted by the corpus luteum during the second half of a woman's cycle (following ovulation). It thickens the lining of the uterus to prepare it to accept implantation of a fertilized egg and to sustain an ongoing pregnancy.

Primary infertility. See infertility, primary.

Prolactin. The hormone produced by the pituitary gland that stimulates production of milk in breastfeeding women. Excessive prolactin levels when a woman is not breastfeeding may result in infertility.

Radiologist. A physician specializing in the use of radiant energy (such as X-rays or fluoroscopes, useful in hysterosalpingograms) for diagnosis and testing.

Reproductive cloning. Taking the genetic material from an "adult cell" (such as blood or skin) and placing it into a human egg from which the nucleus has been removed, then stimulating the cell with electrical current or a chemical solution to "switch on" the proper cells for embryonic growth. After growing to the blastocyst stage, the embryo is transferred to a womb, where the embryo can implant and develop. Such cloning for the purpose of creating a child is illegal in many places; it's considered immoral almost universally.

Reproductive endocrinologist (RE). A subspecialist in ob-gyn with advanced training (a fellowship) in reproductive endocrinology and infertility. While the typical ob-gyn resident receives between five and twelve weeks of training focused on infertility, a fellow spends two to three years specializing in reproductive endocrinology after completion of the ob-gyn residency. Following a year of research and after publishing in a fertility medical journal, the subspecialist becomes board eligible in infertility. Then comes a written test and an oral examination to become a board-certified subspecialist in the field of reproductive endocrinology and infertility. Generally, these highly specialized physicians direct IVF (in vitro fertilization) clinics.

ROSNI (round spermatic nuclear injection). The process of harvesting immature sperm by needle aspiration from the testes. The resulting sperm can be used in the micromanipulation process.

SART. The Society for Assisted Reproductive Technology.

Secondary infertility. See infertility, secondary.

Selective reduction. The termination of one or more fetuses in a multiple pregnancy, leaving the rest to continue to term. The procedure is usually performed between nine and eleven weeks of pregnancy. The term "selective reduction" is sometimes used interchangeably with "multifetal pregnancy reduction." However, some use "selective reduction" to refer only to those pregnancies in which a specific fetus is targeted for reduction because it has been shown to have an abnormality.

Semen. The fluid portion of the ejaculate, consisting of secretions from the seminal vesicles, prostate gland, and several other glands in the male reproductive tract. Semen provides nourishment and protection for the sperm in a medium that allows sperm to travel to a woman's vagina. Semen may also refer to the entire ejaculate, including the sperm.

Semenalysis. A laboratory test used to assess semen quality: sperm quantity, concentration, morphology, and motility. It also measures semen volume and can be used to determine whether infection is present.

Serophene. A brand name for clomiphene citrate.

Sims-Huhner test. See postcoital test (PCT) or Huhner's test.

Sonogram. Image of internal body parts produced by high-frequency sound waves. In the context of infertility treatment, a sonogram is used to detect and count ovarian follicle growth (and disappearance) in many treatments and to detect and monitor pregnancy. Also referred to as ultrasound.

Sonography. The use of ultrasound to create images of internal body parts.

Special revelation. That which God reveals about himself directly, such as through Scripture.

Sperm bank. A place where sperm are kept frozen with liquid nitrogen for later use in artificial insemination.

Sperm count. Also called sperm concentration. The number of sperm in a man's ejaculate, given as the number of sperm per milliliter. The World Health Organization defines a normal sperm count as having 20 million sperm per ejaculate, with 50 percent motility and 60 percent normal morphology (form). The amount of semen in the ejaculation matters, too. If the concentration is less than 20 million sperm per milliliter of ejaculate, it may impair fertility.[1]

Stillbirth. The birth of a dead fetus following the twentieth week of pregnancy.

STD. Sexually transmitted disease.

Sterility. An irreversible condition that prevents conception.

Superovulation. The medication-induced production of exceptional numbers of human ova (eggs) in one menstrual cycle. Also called hyperstimulation.

Surrogate. A woman who becomes pregnant usually by artificial insemination (traditional surrogacy) or surgical transfer of an embryo (gestational surrogacy) for the purpose of carrying the baby to term for another woman.

Testosterone. The male hormone responsible for the formation of secondary sex characteristics (such as deep voice, sperm maturation, facial and body hair) and for supporting the sex drive. Testosterone is also necessary for sperm production.

Therapeutic cloning. Taking the genetic material from an "adult cell" (such as blood or skin) and placing it into a human egg from which the nucleus has been removed, then stimulating the cell with electrical current or a chemical solution to "switch on" the proper cells for embryonic growth. Once the human embryo reaches the blastocyst stage, its embryonic cells are extracted for use in research, thereby killing the embryo. This differs from reproductive cloning in that the embryo is sacrificed for science rather than being created with the goal of transferring it to a woman's womb, where the embryo may implant and develop. Both types of cloning violate several ethical principles.

Thyroid. The endocrine gland located in the neck that produces hormones necessary for fertility.

Traditional surrogacy. See surrogate.

Transfer. Also called embryo transfer (ET). The movement of embryos (whether fresh or thawed from cryopreservation) from a laboratory dish to the uterus following fertilization in an in vitro fertilization (IVF) cycle.

Transvaginal sonogram. A procedure in which a delicately tapered ultrasound probe is inserted into the vagina to generate dramatic, detailed images of the pelvic anatomy. See also ultrasound.

Tubal irrigation. Process of injecting colored dye through the fallopian tubes and observing with a sonogram the movement of fluid to determine if the tubes are open or blocked.

Tubal pregnancy. See ectopic pregnancy.

Ultrasound. In the context of infertility treatment, a procedure in which a picture is displayed on a TV screen by bouncing sound waves off of the internal organs. Often used to monitor follicular development and to examine the fallopian tubes and uterus. Done both abdominally and transvaginally. See also sonography.

Undescended testicles. Failure of the testicles to descend from the abdominal cavity into the scrotum by one year of age. If not repaired by age six, permanent fertility loss may result. Also called cryptorchidism.

Urologist. A physician specializing in the genitourinary tract.

Uterus. The womb. The hollow, muscular organ that houses and nourishes the fetus during pregnancy.

Vagina. The canal leading from the cervix to the outside of a woman's body; the birth passage.

Varicocele (British: varicocoele). An enlarged vein in the scrotum.

Vasectomy reversal. The attempt to restore the flow of sperm through the vas deferens after surgical sterilization.

VIPPS (Verified Internet Pharmacy Practice Sites). A program in which the National Association of Boards of Pharmacy verifies the licensure of online pharmacies.

ZIFT (zygote intrafallopian transfer). A procedure that involves letting egg and sperm "meet" in a laboratory dish. Resulting embryos are then transferred to a healthy fallopian tube, where they can travel to the uterus.

Zygote. A fertilized egg that has not yet divided.

RESOURCES

ORGANIZATIONS

Adoption

Adopt:Assistance, Information, Support: www.adopting.org

Adoption: www.adoption.com

Adoptive Families of America: www.adoptivefamilies.com

National Adoption Information Clearinghouse: www.calib.com/naic

National Council for Adoption: www.ncfa-usa.org

North American Council on Adoptable Children: www.nacac.org

Office of Children's Issues: www.travel.state.gov/adopt.html

RainbowKids: International adoption information:
www.rainbowkids.com

Breastfeeding after Adoption

Website: www.fourfriends.com/abrw/breastfeed.com
Books: Debra Stewart Peterson. *Breastfeeding the Adopted Baby.* San
Antonio, TX: Corona, 1999.
Kathryn Anderson. *Nursing Your Adopted Baby.* Schaumburg, IL: La
Leche League International, 1999.

Childfree Living

Living without Children: www.childfree.net

Embryo Adoption

Embryo Adoption Awareness: www.embryoadoption.org

National Embryo Donation Center: www.embryodonation.org

Snowflakes Embryo Adoption Program: www.snowflakes.org

Infertility Information and Support

While they may not embrace a Christian worldview, the following websites provide information and support for infertility patients.

American College of Obstetricians and Gynecologists (ACOG): www.acog.org

American Infertility Association: www.americaninfertility.org

American Society for Reproductive Medicine (ASRM): www.asrm.org (Provides free abstracts from the journal *Fertility and Sterility*)

Aspire: www.aspire2.com

Bertarelli Foundation: www.bertarelli.edu

Caleb Ministries: www.calebministries.org

Child of My Dreams: www.childofmydreams.com

Conceiving Concepts: www.conceivingconcepts.com

Diethylstilbestrol (DES) and Infertility: www.cdc.gov/DES/

Endometriosis Association: www.endometriosisassn.org

Endometriosis information: www.endozone.org

Ferre Institute infertility project: www.ferre.org

Fertile Thoughts: www.fertilethoughts.net

Fertility Plus: www.fertilityplus.org

Hannah's Prayer Christian Support: www.hannah.org

Infertility resources for consumers: www.ihr.com

InterNational Council on Infertility Information Dissemination, Inc.: www.inciid.com and www.inciid.org

Infertility Awareness Association of Canada: www.iaac.ca/

Infertility and Cancer: www.fertilehope.org

IVF Support: www.ivfconnections.com

Ob-gyn medical information: www.obgyn.net

Polycystic Ovary Syndrome Association (PCOS): www.pcosupport.org

RESOLVE: www.resolve.org

Serono Symposia: www.seronosymposia.org

Stepping Stones: A Ministry of Bethany Christian Services: www.bethany.org/step/

A Torah Infertility Medium of Exchange: www.atime.org

Infertility and Adoption Books

Perspectives Press: www.perspectivespress.com

Tapestry Books: www.tapestrybooks.com

Pregnancy Loss

Center for Loss in Multiple Birth (CLIMB), Inc.: www.climb-support.org

The Compassionate Friends: www.compassionatefriends.org

MEND (Mommies Enduring Neonatal Death): www.mend.org

SHARE Pregnancy and Infant Loss Support: www.nationalshareoffice.com

Surrogacy

Organization of Parents through Surrogacy: www.opts.com

RECOMMENDED BOOKS

Adoption

Patricia Irwin Johnston. *Adopting after Infertility.* Indianapolis, IN: Perspectives Press, 1996.

Gail Steinberg and Beth Hall. *Inside Transracial Adoption.* Indianapolis, IN: Perspectives Press, 2000.

Mary Hopkins-Best. *Toddler Adoption: The Weaver's Craft.* Indianapolis, IN: Perspectives Press, 1998.

Childfree Living

Fact sheet on childfree living available for purchase from RESOLVE's national office, www.RESOLVE.org.

Jean Carter, M.D., and Michael Carter, M.D. *Sweet Grapes: How to Stop Being Infertile and Start Living Again.* Indianapolis, IN: Perspectives Press, 1998.

Christian Perspective of Infertility

Sandra Glahn and William Cutrer, M.D., *When Empty Arms Become a Heavy Burden: Encouragement for Couples Facing Infertility.* Nashville, TN: Broadman and Holman, 1997.

Also Recommended

Debra Bridwell. *The Ache for a Child.* Louisville, CO: MICRA Communications, 1999.

Cindy Dake. *Infertility: A Survival Guide.* Nashville, TN: New Hope, 2002.

Marlo Schalesky. *Empty Womb, Aching Heart.* Minneapolis, MN: Bethany House, 2001.

Parenting after Infertility

Ellen Sarasohn Glazer. *The Long-Awaited Stork.* Lanham, MD: Lexington Books, 1994.

Pregnancy Loss

Maureen Rank. *Free to Grieve: Healing and Encouragement for Those Who Have Experienced the Physical, Mental, and Emotional Trauma of Miscarriage and Stillbirth.* Minneapolis, MN: Bethany House, 1985.

Kathe Wunnenberg. *Grieving the Child I Never Knew.* Grand Rapids: Zondervan, 2001.

Bernadette Keaggy. *A Deeper Shade of Grace.* Bloomington, MN: Bethany House, 1996; and *Losing You Too Soon.* Eugene, OR: Harvest House, 2002.

Secondary Infertility

Harriet Simons. *Wanting Another Child.* Lanham, MD: Lexington Books, 1995.

Third-Party Reproduction

Susan Cooper and Ellen Sarasohn Glazer. *Beyond Infertility: New Paths to Parenthood.* Lanham, MD: Lexington Books, 1994. Chapters on medical treatment and third-party reproduction are comprehensive guides to these complex issues.

RESOLVE provides excellent fact sheets to help couples know what questions to ask their medical teams about these issues, www.RESOLVE.org.

Donor Insemination

Ken Daniels and Erica Haimes, eds. *Donor Insemination: International and Social Science Perspectives.* Melbourne, Australia: Cambridge University Press, 1998.

Egg Donation

Joyce Sutkamp Friedeman. *Building Your Family through Egg Donation.* Fort Thomas, KY: Jolance, 1996.

Sexual Intimacy

William Cutrer, M.D., and Sandra Glahn. *Sexual Intimacy in Marriage.* Grand Rapids: Kregel, 2001.

Doug Rosenau, M.D. *A Celebration of Sex.* Nashville, TN: Nelson, 2002.

Spiritual Crisis

Phillip Yancey. *Disappointment with God.* Grand Rapids: Zondervan, 1988.

Also Recommended

John of the Cross. *Dark Night of the Soul.* New York: Doubleday, Image, 1959.

C. S. Lewis. *The Problem of Pain.* San Francisco: Harper SanFrancisco, 2001.

Henri Nouwen, *The Return of the Prodigal Son.* New York: Doubleday, Image, 1994.

John Piper. *Seeing and Savoring Jesus Christ.* Wheaton, IL: Crossway, 2001.

Evelyn Underhill. *The Spiritual Life.* Harrisburg, PA: Morehouse, 1997.

Notes

Chapter 1. Where We've Been

1. Jeff King, "The Crisis of Infertility" (class paper, Pastoral Care in Human Crises, Southern Baptist Seminary, 2003). Used with permission.

Chapter 2. The Wedded Unmother

1. Abington Urological Specialists, "Infertility: Introduction," 1999, http://www .abington-urology.com/infertility.html.
2. Department of Reproductive Health and Research (RHR), "Infertility," World Health Organization, October 2002, http://www.who.int/reproductive-health/ infertility/index.htm.
3. American Society for Reproductive Medicine, "Patient Fact Sheet: Infertility," ©1997, accessed 16 February 2004, www.asrm.org/Patients/factsheets/infertility -fact.pdf.
4. "Executive Summary of Assisted Reproductive Technologies: Analysis and Recommendations for Public Policy: Infertility." Task Force on Life and the Law, NY State. October 2001. Accessed 16 February 2004, www.health.state.ny.us/hysdoh/ taskfce/execsum.htm.
5. "Quest for Completion: One-Time Moms Facing Secondary Infertility," ABCnews .com, 23 April 2003. Accessed 16 February 2004, abcnews.go.com
6. D. J. Gunnell and P. Ewings. "Infertility Prevalence, Needs Assessment and Purchasing," *Journal of Public Health Medicine (UK)* 16, no. 1 (1994): 29–35.
7. Margaret Renkl, "We Can't Get Pregnant Again," *Parents.com*, 2003, http://www .parents.com/articles/pregnancy/1020.jsp.
8. *1995 National Survey of Family Growth* (Hyattsville, MD: U.S. Department of Health and Human Services, Centers for Disease Control, National Center for Health Statistics, 1997), http://www.cdc.gov/mmwr/preview/mmwrhtml/ss5209a1.htm; as cited in J. C. Abma et al., "Fertility, Family Planning, and Women's Health: New Data from the 1995 National Survey of Family Growth," *Vital and Health Statistics* 23.
9. Centers for Disease Control, "2001 Assisted Reproductive Technology Success Rates," posted 16 December 2003, www.cdc.gov/reproductivehealth/ART01/pref ace. This report is accessible through the authors' website at www.aspire2.com.
10. J. A. Martin, B. E. Hamilton, and S. Ventura , "Births: Preliminary Data for 2000," *National Vital Statistics Report* 49 (Hyattsville, MD: National Center for Health Statistics, 2001), 1–20, as cited in Suzanne C. Tough et al., "Delayed Childbearing and

Its Impact on Population Rate Changes in Lower Birth Weight, Multiple Birth, and Preterm Delivery," *Pediatrics* 100, no. 3 (March 2002), 399-403.

11. "Miscarriage Fact Sheet," March of Dimes Birth Defects Foundation, 2003, http://www.mod.org.

12. Carolyn Coulam, M.D., "Recurrent Pregnancy Loss," *INCIID Insights*, October 2002, www.inciid.org/newsletter/oct/coulam2.html, ©2002, accessed 16 February 2004.

13. "An Infertility Primer," *Harvard Magazine*, 1997, http://www.harvard-maga zine.com.

14. National Center for Health Statistics, as cited in "Study: Men Have Biological Clocks, Too," CNN.com, 6 February 2003, http://www.cnn.com/2003/HEALTH/02/06/male.fertility/.

15. Miranda Devine, "Making a Man Go Father," *Sydney Morning Herald*, 12 January 2003, http://smh.com.au.

16. Sherman Silber, M.D., "Effect of Age on Male Fertility," *Seminars in Reproductive Endocrinology* 9, no. 3 (August 1991), http://www.infertile.com/inthenew/sci/maleage.

17. Emma Ross, "Study Shows Women's Fertility Declines at Age 27, Men's at Age 35," Associated Press, May 1, 2002. For the full text of the Human Reproduction article, see B. Eskenazi et al., "The Association of Age and Semen Quality in Healthy Men," *Human Reproduction* 18, no. 2 (February 2003): 447–54.

18. For example, animal research has shown that a mix of chemicals given to U.S. soldiers during the Gulf War causes degeneration and death of cells, leading to damaged testes and altered sperm production. This may explain why infertility, sexual dysfunction, and other reproductive problems affect many Gulf War veterans. See Mohamed B. Abou-Donia et al., "Testicular Germ-Cell Apoptosis in Stressed Rats Following Combined Exposure to Pyridostigmine Bromide, N, N-Diethyl m-Tolumide (Deet) and Permethrin," *Journal of Toxicology and Environmental Health* 66, no. 1 (10 January 2003), 57–73.

19. "Sperm Defects in Older Men," *BioNews* (Progress Educational Trust) 219, (8 April 2003), http://BioNews.org.uk. See also Rény Slama et al., "Does Male Age Affect the Risk of Spontaneous Abortion?" *American Journal of Epidemiology* 157, no. 9 (May 2003), 815–24. Other research also suggests a link between a man's accelerating age and schizophrenia in his offspring, as well as Apert syndrome, which causes children to be born with distorted skulls and often with webbed fingers or toes.

20. "Ignorance Over Male Infertility," British Broadcasting Corporation, 12 September 1999, http://news.bbc.co.uk/1/hi/health/445018.stm.

21. Abington Urological Specialists, "Infertility: Introduction."

22. "An Infertility Primer."

23. Archibald Hart, Catherine Hart Weber, and Debra Taylor, *Secrets of Eve: Understanding the Mystery of Female Sexuality* (Nashville: Word, 1998), 85.

24. J. E. Norten et al., "Sexual Satisfaction and Functioning in Patients Seeking Infertility Treatment," (paper presented at the annual conference of the American Society for Reproductive Medicine, Orlando, FL, 22 October 2001), cited in "Daily Reproductive Health Report," the Henry J. Kaiser Foundation, KaiserNetwork.org, 22 October 2001.

25. R. P. Barth, D. Brooks, and S. Iyer, "Adoptions in California: Current Demographic Profiles and Projections through the End of the Century" (Berkeley, CA: Child Welfare Research Center, 1995), as cited by National Adoption Information Clearinghouse, http://naic.acf.hhs.gov/pubs/s_infer.cfm.

26. From a variety of sources, including http://www.resolve.org and http://www.adoptivefamilies.com.
27. Patricia Irwin Johnston, *Taking Charge of Infertility* (Indianapolis: Perspectives Press, 1994), 19.
28. Translation by Sandra Glahn. While the qal perfect verb here is often translated "acquire," the *Hebrew and Aramaic Dictionary of the Old Testament* offers "create" as an option.
29. Laurie Tarkan, "Fertility Clinics Begin to Address Mental Health," *New York Times*, 8 October 2002, http://query.nytimes.com/gst/abstract.html?res=F20F1FFD385F0C7B8CDDA90994DA404482.
30. Centers for Disease Control, "2001 Assisted Reproductive Technology Success Rates," *Morbidity and Mortality Weekly Report* 52 (SS–9), 29 August 2003, http://www.cdc.gov/reproductivehealth/ART00/section1.htm.
31. There is little difference by race in the total children born among women aged forty and above; there are, however, appreciable racial differences in the timing of births. See "Childbearing in the United States: What's Going On?" *Population and Development Review*, http://www.popcouncil.org/publications/pdr/usfertility.html.
32. American Society for Reproductive Medicine, "Race Does Not Affect IVF Outcomes," (highlights from the 2002 conference), 15 October 2002, http://www.asrm.org/Media/Press/race.html.
33. Ibid.; Centers for Disease Control, "2001 Assisted Reproductive Technology Success Rates," (SS–9). Results run several years behind because it takes time to gather and collect data after the calendar year has ended, and the live birthrate cannot be calculated until approximately nine months after commencement of a high-tech cycle.
34. Sharon Begley, "The Baby Myth," *Newsweek*, 4 September 1995, 38–45, 47.

Chapter 3. Marital Dynamics

1. C. F. McCartney and C. Y. Wada, "Gender Differences in Counseling Needs during Infertility Treatment," in *Psychiatric Aspects of Reproductive Technology*, ed. N. L. Stotland, (Washington, DC: American Psychiatric Press; 1990).
2. Dan Clements, "A Process of Understanding (for Men)," *RESOLVE of Dallas/Fort Worth Newsletter* (December 1995), 1.
3. Ellen Sarasohn Glazer and Susan Lewis Cooper, *Without Child* (Lexington, MA: Lexington Books, 1988), 3.
4. Carol A. McDonald, "Women and Men Working Together in Management," (lecture, Dallas, Texas, n.d.) labeled it single tracking (men) versus dual tracking (women). Audiocassette #1768, Christian Management Association, Diamond Bar, CA.
5. Debra Tannen, M.D., *You Just Don't Understand: Women and Men in Conversation* (Walkerton, Ontario: Quill, 2001).
6. McDonald, "Women and Men Working Together."
7. Candy Deemer and Nancy Fredericks, "The Woman's Way to Success," *LA Business Journal* (9 October 2002), www.findarticles.com.
8. Elaine Storkey, *The Origins of Difference: The Gender Debate Revisited* (Grand Rapids: Baker Academic, 2001), 84.
9. Aaron R. Kipnis and Elizabeth Herron, "Finding the Battle between the Sexes," *Utne Reader*, January–February 1993, 69–76.

10. The Relationship Institute (Royal Oak, Michigan), "Differences between Men and Women," http://www.relationship-institute.com/freearticles_detail.cfm?article _ID=151.
11. Richard Marrs, M.D., Lisa Friedman Block, and Kathy Kirtland Silverman, *Dr. Richard Marrs' Fertility Book* (New York: Delacorte, 1997), 385–86.
12. Joe McIlhaney, M.D., *1250 Healthcare Questions Women Ask* (Grand Rapids: Baker, 1988), 503.
13. Richard Krusen, "Infertility and Men," *RESOLVE of Dallas/Fort Worth Newsletter*, April–May 1992.
14. Howard J. Markman et al., *Fighting for Your Marriage: Positive Steps for Preventing Divorce and Preserving a Lasting Love* (New York: Jossey-Bass, 2001).
15. Kipnis and Herron, "Finding the Battle between the Sexes," 69–76.
16. A word of caution here: be selective about the support group you choose. Some groups turn into forums for badmouthing doctors and spouses. Also, it's possible to become addicted to cyber relationships at the expense of dealing with reality. The key here is balance.
17. *RESOLVE of Virginia Newsletter*, December 1994, 1.

Chapter 4. Emotional Dynamics

1. Laurie Tarkan, "Fertility Clinics Begin to Address Mental Health," *New York Times*, 9 October 2002, http://www.nytimes.com/2002/10/08/health/psychology/ 08FERT.html.
2. Our book *Sexual Intimacy in Marriage* (Grand Rapids: Kregel, 2001) has a workbook section designed to help you explore a variety of marital issues.
3. Though the study was not extensive enough to reach reliability, a small test group of infertile women in a support group that used yoga, relaxation, and imagery had higher pregnancy rates than a control group and higher rates of spontaneous pregnancy than a standard support group. See A. D. Domar et al., *Fertility and Sterility* 73, no. 4 (2000): 805–11. This study is interesting in its construction and conclusion. Nearly half of the women who started the study stopped participating before its conclusion, so more research is clearly needed.
4. "Support Helps Couples Struggling with Infertility," *Philadelphia Enquirer*, 10 October 2002.
5. According to the American Society for Reproductive Medicine (ASRM), "More than 70 percent of women who are infertile because of body weight disorders will conceive spontaneously if their weight disorder is corrected through a weight-gaining or weight-reduction diet as appropriate. About 12 percent of infertility cases result from extremes in body weight" ("Abnormal Bodyweight," www.protectyourfer tility.com/docs/bodyweight_infertility.doc).

Chapter 6. Where Is God When It Hurts?

1. Elliot Dorff and Aaron Mackler, eds., *Life and Death Responsibilities in Jewish Biomedical Ethics* (New York: Louis Finkelstein Institute, 2000).
2. According to the NET Bible notes, in the ancient Near East, the mandrake was thought to be an aphrodisiac and was therefore used as a fertility drug. The unusual shape of its large forked roots resembles the human body with extended arms and legs. This similarity gave rise to the popular superstition that the mandrake could induce conception. See R. K. Harrison, "The Mandrake and the Ancient World,"

Expositors Quarterly 28 (1956): 188–89; United Bible Societies, *Fauna and Flora of the Bible* (New York: United Bible Societies, 1980), 138–39.

Chapter 7. The Spiritual Struggle

1. Sandra Glahn and William Cutrer, *When Empty Arms Become a Heavy Burden* (Nashville: Broadman and Holman, 1997), 142.
2. Jacqueline Yip Tagawa of Orange Coast Free Methodist Church, Costa Mesa, California.

Chapter 8. The Underlying Question

1. Jan Short, "Infertility Tales," *Self*, May 1989, 191.
2. This is why still today pregnancy dates forty weeks, going back to the first day of the last period. For centuries, people thought women were fertile when they started to bleed.
3. For more about this, see Kenneth Magnuson, "Marriage, Procreation, and Infertility: Reflections on Genesis," *Southern Baptist Journal of Theology* 4, no. 1 (Spring 2000): 26–42.
4. Archibald D. Hart, Catherine Hart Weber, and Debra L. Taylor, *Secrets of Eve: Understanding the Mystery of Female Sexuality* (Nashville: Word, 1998), 100.
5. For a complete treatment of this topic that includes exercises for deepening intimacy, read our book, *Sexual Intimacy in Marriage* (Grand Rapids: Kregel, 2001).

Chapter 9. The Medical Workup

1. Martin Mittelstaedt, "Study Links Male Infertility to Use of Solvent," *Globe and Mail*, 27 February 2003, A6, http://www.kaisernetwork.org/daily_reports. Endocrine-disrupting chemicals (EDCs) such as phthalates, dioxins, and polychlorinated biphenyls have also been linked to reproductive abnormalities and impaired fertility in animals.
2. Survey conducted by the Infertility Awareness Associaton of Canada (IAAC), reported by BBC, 19 September 1999, http://www.news.bbc.co.uk/1/hi/health/445018.stm.
3. Patients can download BBT charts from a variety of sources; to locate these sources, type "BBT chart download" in the search engine.
4. Both urine-based and saliva-based fertility-testing products are available in the U.S. market, though *Newsweek* (19 May 2003) reports that the FDA has not approved many self-test kits due to concerns that patients will substitute self-testing for office-based health care.
5. Linda Carroll, "Sperm May Rely on Heat to Find Egg," Reuters Health, 31 January 2003, http://yalenewhavenhealth.org/HealthNews/reuters/NewsStory0131200310.htm.

Chapter 10. The Continuing Workup

1. Rachel A. Lyons et al., "Peritoneal Fluid, Endometriosis, and Ciliary Beat Frequency in the Human Fallopian Tube," *Lancet* 360, no. 9341 (19 October 2002), 1221–22, as cited in Ed Edelson, "Endometriosis Study Yields Clue to Infertility," *HealthScoutNews Reporter*, 17 October 2002.
2. N. Sinaii et al., "High Rates of Autoimmune and Endocrine Disorders, Fibromyalgia, Chronic Fatigue Syndrome and Atopic Diseases among Women with Endometriosis: A Survey Analysis," *Human Reproduction* 17, no. 10 (October 2002),

2487–781, as cited in Emma Ross, "Endometriosis Study Links Ailments," Associated Press, 26 September 2002.

3. W. P. Dmowski et al., "Cycle-Specific and Cumulative Fecundity in Patients with Endometriosis Who Are Undergoing Controlled Ovarian Hyperstimulation-Intrauterine Insemination or In Vitro Fertilization-Embryo Transfer," *Fertility and Sterility* 78, no. 4 (October 2002): 750–56.

4. General data from John D. Gordon et al., "Recurrent Fetal Loss," *Obstetrics, Gynecology, and Infertility, Handbook for Clinicians*, 5th ed. (Arlington, VA: Scrub Hill Press, 2001), 257.

5. R. P. Dickey et al., *Fertility and Sterility* 78, no. 5 (2002): 1088–95. Among women with ovulatory dysfunction in cycles during which donor sperm was used, additional cycles did further increase the cumulative pregnancy rate.

Chapter 11. The Doctor

1. Center for Advanced Reproductive Services (Farmington, Connecticut) "Frequently Asked Questions," http://www.fertilitycenter-uconn.org/education_faq.htm.

2. "Weight Influences Fertility Treatment," BBC, 24 November 2000 (reporting on information published in the *British Medical Journal*), http://news.bbc.co.uk/1/hi/health/1037056.stm. Extremes of body weight also appear to decrease a woman's chance of getting pregnant through IVF. While normal-weight women became pregnant about half of the time, underweight and overweight women conceived about 35 percent of the time.

3. "Coffee Pregnancy Warning," BBC, 21 February 2003 (reporting on information published in the *British Medical Journal*), www.news.bbc.co.uk/go/em/fr/-/2/hi/health/2780695.stm.

4. Richard R. Ondrizek et al., "The Effect of Commonly Used Herbs on Sperm DNA and Fertilization," *Fertility and Sterility* 71, no. 3 (1999): 517–22.

5. Marritt McKinney, "Lead May Impair Male Fertility: Study," Reuters Health, 6 February 2003.

6. Christine M. Y. Choy et al., "Infertility, Blood Mercury Concentrations and Dietary Seafood Consumption: A Case-Control Study," *British Journal of Obstetrics and Gynaecology: An International Journal of Obstetrics and Gynaecology* 109 (2002): 1121–25.

7. Martin Mittelstaedt, "Study Links Male Infertility to Use of Solvent," *Globe and Mail*, 27 February 2003, A6.

8. Lois Rogers, "Top Perfumes Linked to Cancer Scare Chemical," *London Times*, 24 November 2002.

9. L. J. Burkman, "Marijuana Impacts Sperm Function Both In Vivo and In Vitro: Semen Analyses from Men Smoking Marijuana," (lecture, American Society for Reproductive Medicine conference, San Antonio, 11–15 October 2003), as cited in Daniel DeNoon, "Smoking Marijuana Lowers Fertility: Sperm Burn Out, Less Potent When Men—or Women—Smoke Marijuana," *Web M.D.*, 13 October 2003, http://www.webmd.com/webmddiet/bp/index.html.

10. We explore this subject in greater depth in our forthcoming book *Family Planning* (Grand Rapids: Zondervan, 2005).

11. Frequently cited statistics from the *Journal of Urology* (A. M. Belker, A. J. Thomas Jr., et al., "Results of 1,469 Microsurgical Vasectomy Reversals by the Vasovasostomy Study Group," *Journal of Urology* 145, no. 3 [March 1991]: 505–11) state that the fertility rate decreases as the time between vasectomy and reversal increases. The

pregnancy rate in this study ranged from 67 percent for those with less than three years since the obstruction and 30 percent after 15 or more years of obstruction.

12. Eric Nagourney, "A Study Links Prayer and Pregnancy," *New York Times*, 2 October 2001.

Chapter 12. State of the ARTs

1. Brand names for FSH include Gonal F, Fertinex, Follistim, and Bravelle.
2. One possible option on the horizon that could make fertilization possible without injectables is in vitro maturation, or IVM. A few days before ovulation, as many as thirty to fifty egg follicles have begun to mature, but normally only one will fully ripen for ovulation. If the ova are removed before ovulation, they can be incubated for twenty-eight to thirty-six hours and thus matured in the laboratory. See Mary Duenwald, "25 Years After, New Ideas Are Born in Science of In Vitro Fertilization," *New York Times*, 15 July 2003; and European Society for Human Reproduction and Embryology, abstract no: O–014, www.eurekalert.org/pub_releases/2003-06/esfh -fso062403.php.
3. At the time of this writing, online information about financing infertility treatment is at these sites: http://integramed.com; http://fertilitytreatmentfinancing.com (through HealthReady); and http://amerifee.com/fertility-financing (through Capital One). Patients pursue these options at their own risk.
4. J. A. Collins et al., "An Estimate of the Cost of In Vitro Fertilization Services in the United States in 1995," *Fertility and Sterility* 64 (1995): 538–45.
5. "Drive for Insurance Coverage of Infertility Treatment Raises Questions of Equity, Cost," *The Guttmacher Report on Public Policy* 2, no. 5 (October 1999).
6. Alison McCook, "Insurance Sways Outcome of In Vitro Fertilization," Reuters Health, 28 August 2002; and Tarun Jain, Bernard L. Harlow, and Mark D. Horn- stein, "Insurance Coverage and Outcomes of In Vitro Fertilization," *New England Journal of Medicine*, 29 August 2002.
7. R. T. Burkman et al., "Infertility Drugs and the Risk of Breast Cancer: Findings from the National Institute of Child Health and Human Development Women's Con- traceptive and Reproductive Experiences Study," *Fertility and Sterility* 79, no. 4 (April 2003): 844–51.
8. Merritt McKinney, "No Link Found for Fertility Drugs, Ovarian Cancer," Reuters Health, 24 January 2002, as reported in *American Journal of Epidemiology* (2002): 155.
9. J. Abma et al., "Fertility, Family Planning, and Women's Health: New Data from the 1995 National Survey of Family Growth," *Vital Health Statistics* 23 (1997): 1–114.
10. Rebecca Skloot, "Sally Has Two Mommies and One Daddy," *Popular Science*, March 2003, http://www.popsci.com/popsci/medicine/article/0,12543,411770,00.html.
11. Centers for Disease Control, "2001 Assisted Reproductive Technology Success Rates: National Summary and Fertility Clinic Report," http://www.cdc.gov/repro ductivehealth.art.
12. Ibid.
13. We provide a link to these reports on our website: http://www.aspire2.com.
14. Centers for Disease Control, "2001 Assisted Reproductive Technology Success Rates."
15. "IVF Multiples 'Strain Marriages,'" BBC, 16 October 2003, http://news.bbc.co.uk/1/ hi/health/3196850.stm.

16. F. M. Helmerhorst et al., "Perinatal Outcome of Singletons and Twins after Assisted Conception: A Systematic Review of Controlled Studies," *British Medical Journal* 328 (23 January 2004): 261.

17. The cycle outlined here follows the general format of the University Ob-Gyn Associates of the Fertility Center, connected with the University of Louisville and under the guidance of Dr. Steven Nakajima.

18. For some patients, laparoscopy is required for retrieval (for example, those with cul de sac scarring).

19. It is our belief that every human has the full rights of personhood from the moment life begins.

20. "Nonviable" technically means "not living," but it may also be used to describe those that "can't live" or "in our opinion, won't make it." Patients should ask what their medical team means if they use the term "nonviable." If it means the embryo is still alive but hasn't made the appropriate cell divisions, death is inevitable (and most doctors *would* use "nonviable" for this category). An ethical doctor will be reluctant to transfer embryos that have stopped growing or have failed to reach appropriate milestones. One possibility in such a case is to give the failing embryo a little more time to declare its potential, which often means waiting, using the blastocyst stage as the deciding point of maturity before transferal in questionable cases. Only the hearty will make it. If an embryo is dying, both discarding and transferring are inappropriate. Dignity and respect are always appropriate, and death will inevitably come, usually in a matter of hours.

21. C. S. Pope et al., "Influence of Embryo Transfer Depth on In Vitro Fertilization and Embryo Transfer Outcomes," *Fertility and Sterility* 81, no. 1, 51–58.

22. K. Sharif et al., "Is Prolonged Bed Rest Following Embryo Transfer Useful?" *Fertility and Sterility* 69, no. 3 (1998): 478–81; G. Botta and G. Grudzinskas, "Is a Prolonged Bed Rest Following Embryo Transfer Useful?" *Human Reproduction* 12, no. 11 (November 1997): 2489–92; K. Sharif et al., "Do Patients Need to Remain in Bed Following Embryo Transfer?" *Human Reproduction* 10, no. 6 (June 1995): 1427–29.

23. Advanced Fertility Center of Chicago, "What Is Blastocyst Transfer and How Does That Differ from 2–3 Day Embryo Transfer Techniques?" March 2003, http://www.advanced fertility.com/blastocy.htm.

24. Duenwald, "25 Years After." One researcher has found that the incidence of identical twins, which is only 2 percent among regular IVF pregnancies, is 5.6 percent among pregnancies resulting from blastocyst transfer. Another researcher has observed an even higher incidence, up to 10 percent.

25. R. Schillaci et al., "Vero Cell Effect on In-Vitro Human Blastocyst Development: Preliminary Results," *Human Reproduction* 9 (1994): 1131–35; R. Kaufmann et al., "Cocultured Blastocyst Cryopreservation: Experience of More Than 500 Transfer Cycles," *Fertility and Sterility* 64 (1995): 1125–29; F. Olivennes et al., "Four Indications for Embryo Transfer at the Blastocyst Stage," *Human Reproduction* 9 (1994): 2367–73.

26. B. W. J. Mol, "Cost-Effectiveness of In Vitro Fertilization and Embryo Transfer," *Fertility and Sterility* 73 (2000): 748–54.

27. The chance of having a baby is the same for women in their forties as for women in their twenties if the egg donor is under thirty.

28. Ten years ago, GIFT (gamete intrafallopian transfer; egg and sperm transfer to the tubes) and ZIFT (zygote intrafallopian transfer; one-day-old embryo transfer to the tubes) were popular because IVF laboratories were not able to attain high preg-

nancy rates with longer periods of in vitro culture. Today most programs have abandoned these expensive and invasive tubal procedures and are routinely doing IVF with three-day-old embryo transfers with much improved pregnancy rates.

29. Ramadan Saleh, M.D.,"Increased Sperm Nuclear DNA Damage in Normo-zoospermic Infertile Men: A Prospective Study," *Fertility and Sterility* 78, no. 2 (August 2002), 313–18.

30. Deborah Smith, "Egg and Sperm Race," *Sydney Morning Herald*, 18 November 2002, http://www.smh.com.au/articles/2002/11/17/1037490052866.html.

31. While ROSNI has been shown to result in fertilization and embryo development, those embryos almost never implant, and pregnancies are rare.

32. American Society for Reproductive Medicine, "Studies Show Children of ART Develop Normally," 14 October 2002, http://www.asrm.org/media/press/kids areallright.html.

Chapter 13. A Moral Minefield

1. Because the events surrounding fertilization happen so closely to each other, it's fine to say that life begins at fertilization. To be technically correct, however, we specify life as beginning when DNA aligns, as in cloning eggs there is no "moment of fertilization" yet there is the beginning of human life.

2. For a more thorough exploration of this subject, see Robert Pyne, *Humanity and Sin: The Creation, Fall and Redemption of Humanity* (Nashville: Word, 1999). Of particular interest is chapter 5, "The Immaterial Aspect of Human Nature."

3. During the first critical days of embryonic development, three children were grown on pieces of cow uterus before being transferred to their mother's womb—a treatment so controversial that it's now viewed by the FDA and many scientists as experimentation on unborn children. If this so-called co-culture method were to be used today, the FDA would want any offspring tracked for life and forbidden to donate blood or organs out of fear that they might transmit mad cow disease or some yet unknown cross-species virus. (Rebecca Skloot, "Sally Has Two Mommies and One Daddy," *Popular Science*, March 2003.) Because ART has proceeded largely without formal oversight, sometimes—such as in situations such as this—it is difficult to determine a risk/benefit ratio with any sort of accuracy.

4. Leon Kass, M.D., quoted in Robin Marantz Henig, "Think Baby Louise, and Don't Be Afraid," *Washington Post*, Sunday, 13 July 2003, B1. President George W. Bush appointed Dr. Kass as his administration's leading bioethics adviser.

5. During the early days of the national debate over embryonic stem cell research, the press noted that a group of senators known for their strong pro-life positions urged the president to approve federal funding for research on human embryos. Five of these senators are members of the Church of Jesus Christ of Latter-Day Saints, and their views on embryos are based on Mormon teaching regarding ensoulment. Mormon philosophy holds that the unimplanted blastocysts haven't yet been animated by the human spirit. See "Stem Cell Research, Morality, and Law" at Dallas Seminary's website, http://dts.edu/publications/kindredspirit/article.aspx?id =124 for more information.

6. The American College of Obstetricians and Gynecologists' *Obstetric-Gynecologic Terminology* (ed. Edward C. Hughes [Philadelphia: F. A. Davis, 1972) defined conception as the implantation of the blastocyst, stating that it was not synonymous with fertilization.

Chapter 14. Determining Right from Wrong

1. Tom Beauchamp and James Childress, *Principles of Biomedical Ethics*, 5th ed. (New York: Oxford University Press, 2001).
2. Autonomy can be compromised if physicians pressure patients to do procedures with which they are uncomfortable (such as transferring more embryos than they wish or cryopreserving embryos). Patients must be conscious that their own hesitation to question or disagree with their doctors can compromise autonomy. In addition, husbands and wives must give each other full freedom to limit their treatment options so that all options fall within ethical parameters that are comfortable to both spouses.
3. This principle is presented in *Instruction on Respect for Human Life in Its Origin and on the Dignity of Procreation (Donum Vitae)*, from the Vatican Congregation for the Doctrine of the Faith (1987). Available online at http://www.vatican .va/roman_curia/congregations/cfaith/documents/rc_con_cfaith_doc_19870222 _respect-for-human-life_en.html.
4. Since January 1991, under German law, a maximum of three embryos can be transferred to a woman's uterus, but only as many female eggs (oocytes) can be fertilized as are planned to be transferred, and then they all have to be transferred in one go, regardless of quality, because embryo selection and storage by freezing is forbidden. Only freezing of oocytes in the pronuclear stage is allowed, which means that selection has to be performed at that stage of development and not later. See European Society for Human Reproduction and Embryology, "ART Laws Put Patients at Risk and Should Be Changed, Warns Head of Germany's IVF Registry," press release, http://eurekalert.org/pub_releases/2003–06/esfh-alp062403.php.
5. We know from blood tests that approximately half of all pregnancies end in miscarriage. Often the mother is never even aware of the conception.
6. In the past, some clinics were more apt to transfer large numbers of embryos and rely on multifetal pregnancy reduction as a backup procedure if numerous embryos implanted. Other clinics, concerned with the ethics of this practice, chose to transfer lower numbers of embryos. While they have been vindicated by the higher success rates that have come with transferring lower numbers of embryos, the challenge now is that clinics seeking better success rates will often still fertilize numerous embryos but discard those of "lesser quality." The challenge is to limit not only the number transferred but also the number created. While success rates may turn out to be lower, the ethics of discarding embryos must be considered.
7. The European strategy of transferring only one embryo per fertilization cycle "has been shown to be as effective as transferring more than one, as long as the couple goes through at least two cycles. American doctors say that practice is unrealistic in this country, where most insurance companies do not pay for IVF." Mary Duenwald, "25 Years After, New Ideas Are Born in Science of In Vitro Fertilization," *New York Times*, 15 July 2003.
8. Stem cells are "unspecialized cells that renew themselves for long periods through cell division." Under certain "physiologic or experimental conditions, they can be induced to become cells with special functions." For more information, go to the National Institutes of Health website: http://stemcells.nih.gov.
9. While it was initially argued that embryonic stem cells were essential for developing promising therapies to cure diseases such as Alzheimer's and Parkinson's, further research is indicating that adult stem cells (an approach to finding cures for diseases that does not require the destruction of human embryos) are turning out

to be more versatile than once thought. For current information about this, check out the Center for Bioethics and Human Dignity website: http://www.cbhd.org.

10. American Society for Reproductive Medicine, "Preimplantation Genetic Diagnosis May Be More Useful in Some Cases Than in Others: Women Who Have Experienced Recurrent Pregnancy Loss Seem to Benefit the Most," press release, 16 October 2002. Available online at http://www.asrm.org/Media/Press/genetictech.html.

11. Paul McKeague, "Screening of Embryos a Growing Trend," *Ottawa Citizen*, 10 March 2003.

Chapter 15. Three's Company

1. InterNational Council on Infertility Information Dissemination, "Statement from Dr. Cappy Rothman, Medical Director of California Cryobank, regarding Gross Irresponsibility of Human Egg Auction," PR Newswire, 26 October 1999, http://www.inciid.org/fertinews/eggauction1.html.

2. David Plotz, "The Myths of the Nobel Sperm Bank," *MSN Slate Magazine*, 23 February 2001.

3. For a transcript of the Oprah Winfrey show on this topic, go to http://www.oprah.com/tows/pastshows/200305/tows_past_20030522.jhtml.

4. Simone Bateman Novaes, "The Medical Management of Donor Insemination," in Ken Daniels and Erica Haimes, eds., *Donor Insemination: International and Social Science Perspectives* (Melbourne, Australia: Cambridge University Press, 1998), 109.

5. Richard Willing, "U.S. Sperm Banks to Give Gift of Life to the U.K.," *USA Today*, 14 August 2002.

6. Genesis Fertility Centre (Vancouver, B.C., Canada), "Male Infertility Services," http://www.genesis-fertility.com/services/services10.htm. Accessed 19 February 2004.

7. Consider the language of 1 Timothy 3:2 requiring that elders be the "husband of but one wife" compared with the parallel idea for widows in 1 Timothy 5:9 (see KJV and NASB translations), "having been the wife of one man." Whether this means "faithful to one's spouse" or "having only one spouse," both suggest a singular relationship rather than a plurality of spouses.

8. Robert Chisholm, (Hebrew class lecture, Dallas Theological Seminary, spring 2001).

9. Paul Bender, *J Vibrations*, no. 8, http://www.jvibe.com/jvibrations/issue8/responsa2.shtml.

10. Norman L. Geisler, *Christian Ethics* (Grand Rapids: Baker, 1990), 187.

11. Bender, *J Vibrations*.

12. The translators' notes in the NET Bible (http://www.bible.org) point out: "The phrase 'one flesh' occurs only here and must be interpreted in light of v. 23. There the man declares that the woman is bone of his bone and flesh of his flesh. To be one's 'bone and flesh' is to be related by blood to someone. For example the phrase describes the relationship between Laban and Jacob (Gen 29:14); Abimelech and the Shechemites (Judg 9:2; his mother was a Shechemite); David and the Israelites (2 Sam 5:1); David and the elders of Judah (2 Sam 19:12); and David and his nephew Amasa (2 Sam 19:13, see 2 Sam 17:2; 1 Chr 2:16–17). The expression 'one flesh' seems to indicate that they become, as it were, 'kin,' at least legally (a new family unit is created) or metaphorically. In this first marriage in human history, the woman was literally formed from the man's bone and flesh."

13. Brian Calhoun, M.D., *When a Husband Is Infertile* (Grand Rapids: Baker, 1994), 92–93.
14. Bender, *J Vibrations*.

Chapter 16. Aid in the Begetting

1. The American Society for Reproductive Medicine issued guidelines in 1997 that egg donors should be under thirty-four years old. An extensive study suggests, however, that this age should be lowered to thirty-two or under. See Faber et al., "The Impact of an Egg Donor's Age and Her Prior Fertility on Recipient Pregnancy Outcome," *Fertility and Sterility* 68 (1997): 370–72.
2. American Society for Reproductive Medicine, "Fertility Experts Discuss New Research Findings at ASRM Annual Meeting in Seattle," press release, 14 October 2002, http://www.asrm.org.
3. Sharon Kirkey, "Nobody's Child: Like Adoptees, Donor-Conceived Offspring Are Demanding Identifying Information," *Ottawa Citizen*, 3 March 2003. For women in their forties, DE success rates were significantly higher than those of nondonor cycles.
4. Vatican English language text of "Instruction on Respect for Human Life in Its Origin and on the Dignity of Procreation: Replies to Certain Questions of the Day," issued on 22 February 1987 by the Congregation for the Doctrine of the Faith, published 10 March 1987. Available online at http://www.vatican.va/roman_curia/congregations/cfaith/documents/rc_con_cfaith_doc_19870222_respect-for-human-life_en.html.
5. "In Vitro Fertilization" statement by Christian Medical and Dental Associations, 13 May 1983. Available at www.cmds.org.
6. American Society for Reproductive Medicine, "Fertility Experts Discuss New Research Findings."
7. Henry J. Kaiser Family Foundation, "Reproductive Health Services: Fertility Experts Discuss New Research Findings at ASRM Annual Meeting in Seattle," 17 October 2002, http://www.kaisernetwork.org/daily_reports/rep_index.cfm?DR_ID=14092, Nov 9, 2002.
8. Alan Mozes, "Third of U.S. Egg Donors Unwilling to Donate Again," Reuters Health, 7 July 2003, http://12.31.13.115/HealthNews/reuters/NewsStory070220035.htm.
9. "Surrogate Sues Parents over Unborn Twins," *CNN.com*, 13 August 2001, http://www.cnn.com.
10. See appendix 2 for the Christian Medical Association's complete statement on reproductive technology.
11. Nicholas Wade, "Clinics Hold More Embryos Than Had Been Thought," *New York Times*, 9 May 2003; Stuart Shepard, "Frozen Embryo Adoption on the Rise," Family News in Focus, http://www.family.org. At the time of this writing, it is estimated that nine thousand frozen embryos are available for adoption.
12. Gabor T. Kovacs et al., "Embryo Donation at an Australian University In-Vitro Fertilisation Clinic: Issues and Outcomes," *Medical Journal of Australia* 178, no. 3 (3 February 2003): 127–29. This finding is based on data gathered from Melbourne's Monash University IVF clinic between January 1991 and July 2002. Of 1,246 couples who relinquished frozen embryos, 89.5 per cent (1,116) discarded them rather than choosing to donate. Ninety-eight couples were on a waiting list for donated embryos.
13. Randy Alcorn, "Are Frozen Embryos Persons Worthy of Protection?" Eternal Perspectives Ministries, http://www.epm.org/frozen.html. Accessed 19 February 2004.

14. Essex Fertility Center, "Embryo Cryopreservation," http://www.essexfertility.co .uk/pages/freeze.htm.
15. In general, "survival" means more than half of the embryo's cells are viable. Presently only about one-third of the thawed embryos have 100 percent cell survival. Be sure to check both the embryo thaw-survival rate and the live birthrate for any clinic you're considering.
16. "Frozen Embryos Increase Ectopic Risk," *Telegraph Group Limited*, 15 October 2003, http://www.telegraph.co.uk/health/main.jhtml?xml=/health/2003/10/15/wfert 15.xml. A team from Brown University compared the outcomes of 2,844 IVF cycles. Of those, 2,452 used fresh embryos, while 392 were frozen embryos. Nine out of 490 fresh-embryo pregnancies, or less than 2 percent, were ectopic, but 6 out of the 19 frozen-embryo pregnancies implanted outside the womb.
17. The single greatest obstacle to embryo adoption is abortion advocacy. Any act that could be interpreted as increasing moral respect or providing legal protection for the human embryo is feared to be an assault on abortion rights, according to Paige Comstock Cunningham, "Embryo Adoption or Embryo Donation? The Distinction and Its Implications," Center for Bioethics and Human Dignity, http://www .cbhd.org/resources/reproductive/cunningham_2003–04–17.htm.
18. The National Embryo Donation Center is endorsed by the Christian Medical Association. For more information, go to http://www.embryoadoptions.org.
19. Excerpted from the English translation of the Donum Vitae (Congregation for the Doctrine of the Faith), "Instruction on Respect for Human Life in Its Origin and on the Dignity of Procreation: Replies to Certain Questions of the Day," http://www.seminarianlifelink.org/biotechnology/donumvitae.htm.
20. Note that this is per transfer and excludes embryos that do not survive freezing and thawing.
21. Centers for Disease Control, "2001 Assisted Reproductive Technology Success Rates," http://www.cdc.gov/nccdphp/drh/art.htm. The annual update of this report is accessible through our website, http://www.aspire2.com.
22. Associated Press, "Twelve Years Old at Birth," *Globe and Mail*, 4 February 2002.

Chapter 17. Using a Donor

1. Bill Cordray, Donor Conception Network, http://freespace.virgin.net/dcnet.web site/ARTICLES/Bill.htm.
2. Debra Evans, *Without Moral Limits* (Westchester, IL: Crossway, 1989), 121.
3. Tamara Traubmann and Haim Shadmi, "Couple Allowed to Choose Baby's Gender to Avoid Halakhic Dilemma," *Haaretz Daily*, 18 October 2002.
4. Sharon Kirkey, "Nobody's Child: Like Adoptees, Donor-Conceived Offspring Are Demanding Identifying Information," *Ottawa Citizen*, 3 March 2003.
5. Cindy Marie Mack, letter to the editor, *Maclean's Magazine*, 10 June 2002.
6. "Children of a Lesser Dad" *Sydney Morning Herald*, 20 December 2002, http://www.smh.com.au/text/articles/2002/12/20/1040174389982.htm.
7. Ibid.

Chapter 18. Loss upon Loss

1. Hannah's Prayer (http://www.hannah.org) has an excellent list of resources for couples facing this type of loss.
2. Philip M. Boyce, John T. Condon and David A. Ellwood, "Pregnancy Loss: A Major Life Event Affecting Emotional Health and Well-Being," *Medical Journal of Australia* 176, no. 6 (18 March 2002), 250–51.

3. Ronald Green, "Determining Moral Status," *Bioethics.net* (MIT Press), 2002, http://bioethics.net/hottopics/stemcells/excerpts_green.php?page=4.

4. Ronald F. Feinberg, M.D., "Pregnancy Loss: Approaches to Evaluation and Treatment," *Yale–New Haven Medical Center*, 19 November 1997, http://www.med.yale.edu/obgyn/kliman/pages/Feinberg/Pregloss.html.

5. The National Stillbirth Society, "Frequently Asked Questions about Stillbirth," http://www.stillnomore.org.

6. Feinberg, "Pregnancy Loss."

7. Ibid.

8. Rebecca Smith Waddell, "Recurrent Pregnancy Loss Testing," *Fertility Plus*, 10 July 2001, http://www.fertilityplus.org/faq/miscarriage/rpl.html.

9. Edward Lyons, M.D., "Ectopic Pregnancy—New and Useful Sonographic Signs," *Topics in Ultrasonography*, March 2003.

10. J. Bouyer et al., "Risk Factors for Ectopic Pregnancy: A Comprehensive Analysis Based on a Large Case-Control, Population-Based Study in France" *American Journal of Epidemiology* 157, no. 3 (1 February 2003): 185–94.

11. Ibid.

12. L. A. Schieve et al., "Spontaneous Abortion among Pregnancies Conceived Using Assisted Reproductive Technology in the United States," *Obstetrics and Gynecology* 101 (2003): 959–67, cited in "Assisted Reproduction May Not Up Miscarriage Rate," Reuters Health, 1 May 2003.

Chapter 19. Infertility Patient as Parent

1. "Quest for Completion: One-Time Moms Facing Secondary Infertility," ABC.com, 23 April 2003, http://abcnews.go.com, accessed 19 Febuary 2004. Within the last decade, over 3.3 million Americans who reported having impaired fertility had at least one child, according to the American Society for Reproductive Medicine. www.asrm.org.

2. *1995 National Survey of Family Growth* (Hyattsville, MD: U.S. Department of Health and Human Services, Centers for Disease Control, National Center for Health Statistics, 1997), http://www.cdc.gov/mmwr/preview/mmwrhtml/ss5209a1.htm; cited in J. C. Abma et al., "Fertility, Family Planning, and Women's Health: New Data from the 1995 National Survey of Family Growth," *Vital Health Statistics* 23.

3. Karen Steiner, "The Only Child," *KidSource Online*, http://www.kidsource.com/kidsource/content2/only.child.html.

4. Anna Hjelmstedt et al., "Personality Factors and Emotional Responses to Pregnancy among IVF Couples in Early Pregnancy: A Comparative Study," *Acta Obstetricia et Gynecologica Scandinavica* 82, no. 2 (February 2003), 152.

5. Depression caused by factors such as lack of sleep, stress, and unmet expectations happens to fathers as well as to mothers, both in birth and adoption. In fact, more than 65 percent of mothers who adopted internationally experience postadoption depression. Harriet McCarthy, "Post Adoption Depression," Rainbow Kids, www.rainbowkids.com/articles/800postdepression.htm, accessed 19 February 2004.

6. Jennifer Frey, "Parenting after Infertility: How It Changes Your Approach," Disney Online's Family Fun, http://www.familyfun.go.com/raisingkids/baby/care/feature/dony57infertility/dony57infertility.html.

Chapter 20. Resolution

1. Dan Clements, "Stop in the Name of Love," *RESOLVE of Dallas/Fort Worth Newsletter*, fall 1993, 1. Mr. Clements is the former chair of RESOLVE, Inc.
2. Mark T. McDermott, "Overview of Independent or Private Adoption," http://www.theadoptionadvisor.com/independent.html.
3. Karen Spar, *Foster Care and Adoption Stats*, Congressional Research Service report for Congress, prepared at the request of the House Subcommittee on Human Resources, Casanet.org (Court-Appointed Special Advocate), 15 January 1997, http://www.casanet.org/library/foster-care/fost.htm.
4. Victor Groza, M.D., and Daniela F. Ileana, "Preparing Families for Adoption of Instiutionalized Children with Special Needs and/or Children at Risk for Special Needs," http://www.comeunity.com/adoption/special_needs/groza-issues.html.
5. Nancy Gibbs, "Making Time for a Baby," *Time*, 15 April 2002.
6. "Couples in Pre-Kid, No-Kid Marriages Happiest" *USA Today*, 12 August 1997.
7. James Orr, ed., *International Standard Bible Encyclopedia* (Grand Rapids: Eerdmans, 1939).

Appendix 1. Workbook

1. Based on the research presented in Howard Markman et al., *Fighting for Your Marriage: Positive Steps for Preventing Divorce and Preserving a Lasting Love* (New York: Jossey-Bass, 2001).
2. J. E. Norten et al., "Sexual Satisfaction and Functioning in Patients Seeking Infertility Treatment," (paper presented at the annual conference of the American Society for Reproductive Medicine, Orlando, FL, 22 October 2001), cited in "Daily Reproductive Health Report," the Henry J. Kaiser Foundation, KaiserNetwork.org, 22 October 2001.
3. Erma Bombeck, "Pat," *Motherhood the Second Oldest Profession* (New York: McGraw Hill, 1983).

Glossary

1. Mark Perloe, M.D., "Will Abstaining Improve Sperm Count?" iVillage: the Internet for Women, 6 July 1998, http://ivillage.com, accessed 19 February 2004.

INDEX

Italicized page numbers indicate references to illustrations.

laparoscopy *(continued)*
  development of, 18
lasers, 130
Leah, 77, 79–81
legacy, spiritual, 250–51
Levirate marriage, 187–88, 276
LH. *see* luteinizing hormone (LH)
libido, problems with, 115
life, beginning of, 164
loneliness, 47
loss. *see also* grief; mourning
  of a child, 19
  feelings of, 48
  and pregnancy, 219–40
lovemaking, 99–100. *see also* sex
  and sex, 107
LPD (luteal phase defect), 277
lubricants, 141
Lupron, 166, 277
lupus, 124
luteal phase, 277
luteal phase defect (LPD), 277
luteinizing hormone (LH), 119, 145, *146*,
  147, 276

male infertility, 135
  increase of, 112
mandrake, 80, 292n. 2
manhood
  sense of, 37
  threat to, 113
manual sex, 104. *see also* masturbation
marriage
  biblical description of, 189
  de-stressing, 43–45
  exercises, 257
  goal of, 103
  in human history, 299n. 12
  and infertility, 35–45
  and intimacy, 238
  Levirate, 187–88, 276
  purpose of, 106
  strengthening, 52
  and third-party donors, 210
  unity of, 197
Mary, icons of, 83
masculinity, 37
masturbation. *see also* manual sex
  defined, 277
  and specimen collection, 114

McIlhaney, Joe, 188
medical care
  ethical issues of, 19
  managing, 53
medical expenses, 73
medical records, copies of, 137
medical treatment. *see* treatment
medical workup, 109–20
medications, 145
  and cancer, 149
  causing infertility, 112
  changing, 115
  for ovulation, 126
  and treatment, 14
medicine, art of, 19
men
  and aging, 25
  and compartmental thinking, 38
  and conversation, 40
  effects of infertility on, 26
  and fertility problems, 112
  and pressure, 100
Menning, Barbara Eck, 239
menopause, premature, 25
menstrual cycle, 277
  history of, 111
  irregular, 118
  normal, 117
menstrual pain, 124
mercury, 139
MESA (microscopic epididymal sperm
  aspiration), 157, 173, 277
messenger hormones, 119–20, 127, 146,
  151
methotrexate, 224–26, 277
metphormin, 125, 277. *see also* Glucophage
Metrodin, 148, 277
Michal, 76
micromanipulation, 18, 156–57, 278
microscopes, 18
microscopic epididymal sperm aspiration
  (MESA), 157, 173, 277
Miller, Calvin, 77
Milophene, 14, 119, 278. *see also* clomiphene
  citrate
mind-body connection, 27–28
miscarriage, 19, 219–24
  and age, 154, 221
  defined, 278
  and infertility, 24

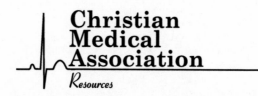

**Christian
Medical
Association**
Resources

Medically reliable ... biblically sound. That is the promise of Christian Medical Association *Resources* and our publishing partnership with Zondervan. Because your health is at stake, you cannot settle for anything less than the whole truth.

From these resources, people's faith can draw from both the knowledge of medical science and the wisdom of God's word. You will benefit from the cutting-edge knowledge of experienced, trusted, and respected doctors. These persons of faith and science can help you gain new insights into the vital link between health and spirituality. A sound biblical analysis of treatments and technologies is essential to protecting yourself from seemingly harmless — yet spiritually, ethically, or medically unsound — options.

Founded in 1931, the Christian Medical Association helps thousands of doctors minister to their patients by imitating the Great Physician, Jesus Christ. The Christian Medical Association provides a voice on the important bioethical issues of our time to the public, the media, and our policy makers. We minister to needy patients around the world through medical missions. We evangelize and disciple the next generation of Christian doctors via campus ministries on nearly every medical and dental school. And, we provide educational and inspirational resources to the church.

To learn more about the Christian Medical Association and its sister organization, the Christian Dental Association, browse the website at *www.cmda.org* or call Christian Medical & Dental Associations' Life & Health Resources at 888-231-2637.

"Dear friend, I pray that you may enjoy good health and that all may go well with you, even as your soul is getting along well."

3 John 2

Share Your Thoughts

With the Author: Your comments will be forwarded to the author when you send them to *zauthor@zondervan.com*.

With Zondervan: Submit your review of this book by writing to *zreview@zondervan.com*.

Free Online Resources at

www.zondervan.com

Zondervan AuthorTracker: Be notified whenever your favorite authors publish new books, go on tour, or post an update about what's happening in their lives at www.zondervan.com/authortracker.

Daily Bible Verses and Devotions: Enrich your life with daily Bible verses or devotions that help you start every morning focused on God. Visit www.zondervan.com/newsletters.

Free Email Publications: Sign up for newsletters on Christian living, academic resources, church ministry, fiction, children's resources, and more. Visit www.zondervan.com/newsletters.

Zondervan Bible Search: Find and compare Bible passages in a variety of translations at www.zondervanbiblesearch.com.

Other Benefits: Register yourself to receive online benefits like coupons and special offers, or to participate in research.

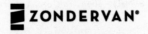

◢ ZONDERVAN®

ZONDERVAN.com/
AUTHORTRACKER
follow your favorite authors